Clinical Management of Insomnia

First Edition

Karl Doghramji, MD
Professor of Psychiatry and Human Behavior
Jefferson Medical College
Director, Sleep Disorders Center
Thomas Jefferson Hospital
Philadelphia, Pa

Paul P. Doghramji, MD
Attending Physician
Collegeville Family Practice
Collegeville, Pa

D1447342

NAL
COMMUNICATIONS, INC.

Important safety information

Rozerem™ (ramelteon) is indicated for the treatment of insomnia characterized by difficulty with sleep onset. Rozerem can be prescribed for long-term use. Rozerem should not be used in patients with hypersensitivity to any components of the formulation, severe hepatic impairment, or in combination with fluvoxamine. Failure of insomnia to remit after a reasonable period of time should be medically evaluated, as this may be the result of an unrecognized underlying medical disorder. Hypnotics should be administered with caution to patients exhibiting signs and symptoms of depression. Rozerem has not been studied in patients with severe sleep apnea, severe COPD, or in children or adolescents. The effects in these populations are unknown. Avoid taking Rozerem with alcohol. Rozerem has been associated with decreased testosterone levels and increased prolactin levels. Health professionals should be mindful of any unexplained symptoms possibly associated with such changes in these hormone levels. Rozerem should not be taken with or immediately after a high-fat meal. Rozerem should be taken within 30 minutes before going to bed and activities confined to preparing for bed. The most common adverse events seen with Rozerem that had at least a 2% incidence difference from placebo were somnolence, dizziness, and fatigue. Please see enclosed prescribing information.

Published by
Professional Communications, Inc.

Marketing Office:
400 Center Bay Drive
West Islip, NY 11795
(t) 631/661-2852
(f) 631/661-2167

Editorial Office:
PO Box 10
Caddo, OK 74729-0010
(t) 580/367-9838
(f) 580/367-9989

For orders only, please call
1-800-337-9838
or visit our website at
www.pcibooks.com

ISBN 13: 978-1-932610-14-7
ISBN 10: 1-932610-14-6

Printed in the United States of America

DISCLAIMER
The opinions expressed in this publication reflect those of the authors. However, the authors make no warranty regarding the contents of the publication. The protocols described herein are general and may not apply to a specific patient. Any product mentioned in this publication should be taken in accordance with the prescribing information provided by the manufacturer.

This text is printed on recycled paper.

DEDICATION

This book is dedicated to our families for their endless love, support, and encouragement.

ACKNOWLEDGMENT

I would like to knowledge my wife, Kathleen, for her firm support that was always abundant wind in my sails during this project; Karl, whose encouragement and guidance are more than a brother could ever ask from a brother; and my colleagues and coworkers, whose help in the office is above and beyond what one could expect.

—PPD

TABLE OF CONTENTS

TABLES

FIGURES

vii

1 Introduction

Sleep takes up one third of our life. The public's view of sleep has ranged from an enjoyable and desirable state to a waste of time; the latter view is often shared by physicians.[1] This trivialization of sleep is evident in a trend over the past century: to spend as much time awake as possible at the expense of losing sleep, seeking more than 18 hours of wakefulness—thus we "borrow" from the time we would normally spend sleeping. And we do this believing one of the following: that there are no consequences, that the consequences are negligible or tolerable, or that what is borrowed can always be paid back at some later date, eg, a weekend. With the advent of more and more ways to stay awake, and more and more reasons to stay awake, many of us are drawn into sleep deprivation.

But insomnia is not sleep deprivation. It is the inability to sleep even when given ample opportunity to do so. The "cure" for sleep deprivation is to simply get more sleep, but treatment is not so simple for insomnia. A staggering 10% to 20% of all Americans and the majority of primary care patients express this sleep complaint. Even though insomnia can exist as an independent disorder, it is most often the consequence of an existing medical or psychiatric problem. Therefore, in clinical settings, it offers a most valuable clue to the etiology of the patient's underlying problem. As in the case of sleep deprivation, we are discovering that lessened sleep amount and/or quality due to insomnia has consequences as well. For example, a patient whose sleep is interrupted by frequent awakenings and arousals as a result of nocturia can develop impairments in next-day functioning due to the sleep fragmentation.

Thus it behooves the primary care clinician to understand sleep and the nature and causes of its disruption. When sleep is normal, the patient is usually better off. When sleep is disturbed, its details offer important information into the understanding of the nature of underlying medical and psychiatric illnesses. Sleep disruption itself can cause decrements in the patient's quality of life, contribute to overall morbidity, and may even be associated with premature death. The clinician should have a high index of suspicion of its existence and raise the level of urgency in treating it.

This book is intended to instruct the primary care practitioner on the most salient issues surrounding the most common complaint regarding sleep, insomnia. We will examine normal sleep processes, discuss how to identify abnormal sleep, and, once identified, how to embark on the path of rectifying the problem and restoring normal sleep function.

REFERENCE

1. Harvey AG. Insomnia: symptom or diagnosis? *Clin Psychol Rev.* 2001;21:1037-1059.

2
Normal Sleep

Sleep comprises one third of our adult life. It is essential for normal functioning; without it, we experience memory lapses, have difficulty with concentration, experience mood alterations, become more prone to accidents, perform poorly at work, and experience breaches in interpersonal relationships.[1,2] Animals deprived of sleep will experience metabolic abnormalities and eventually die.[3] Despite all of this information, however, we do not understand the *why's* of sleep. Scientists have yet to determine how physical and psychological restorative processes are coordinated during sleep and why such a behaviorally disconnected state is necessary to accomplish these tasks.

From a behavioral standpoint, sleep is characterized by diminished responsiveness to, and perceptual disengagement from, the environment. In these ways, it is similar to coma, with the exception that it is readily reversible. However, from a neurophysiologic standpoint, it bears no resemblance to this state at all. During sleep, the brain is highly active and undergoes characteristic changes that translate into parallel changes, not just in the central nervous system, but throughout the body. The apparent quiescence of the sleeper is a product of active processes that diminish responsiveness to environmental stimuli. At the same time, there is a perceptual disengagement from the environment. However, this disengagement is not complete when important environmental sensory information is monitored, again emphasizing the active nature of the brain during sleep. An example is the mother who responds to the infant's whimper, yet sleeps through other loud noises of lesser significance.[4]

Decades of sleep research have confirmed Aesrinsky and Kleitman's original discovery of rapid eye movement (REM) sleep in 1953 and have conclusively demonstrated that sleep is comprised of two fundamentally distinct states, REM and non-REM sleep, which repeat in cyclical fashion throughout the night, forming a pattern widely known as sleep architecture (**Figure 2.1**). Proper characterization of sleep stages necessitates the simultaneous monitoring of the numerous physiologic parameters, a process known as polysomnography. Minimally required are the electro-encephalogram (EEG), electro-oculogram (EOG), and electromyogram (EMG) of skeletal muscle, usually the submentalis. Patterns for each of these parameters during the sleep of a young adult are depicted in **Figures 2.2 through 2.7**.

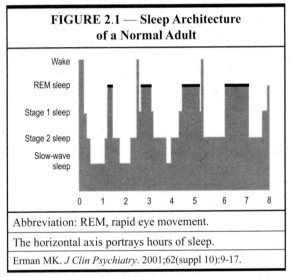

FIGURE 2.1 — Sleep Architecture of a Normal Adult

Abbreviation: REM, rapid eye movement.

The horizontal axis portrays hours of sleep.

Erman MK. *J Clin Psychiatry*. 2001;62(suppl 10):9-17.

The relative distribution of sleep stages changes with age (**Figure 2.8**). Delta sleep is maximal in children and diminishes markedly with age, especially during adolescence. Seniors may have little or no

FIGURE 2.2 — Polysomnography of Patient Who Is Awake

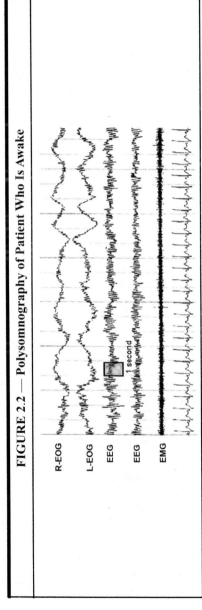

Abbreviations: EEG, electroencephalogram; EMG, electromyogram; L-EOG, left electro-oculogram; R-EOG, right electro-oculogram.

In this awake patient, >50% of each epoch contains α activity. Slow rolling eye movements or eye blinks will be seen in the EOG channels. Relatively high submental EMG muscle tone is evident.

Illustrated Guide to Polysomnography: Normal Sleep, CD-ROM. Available at: http://aasmnet.org/SleepEdSeries.aspx. Accessed December 13, 2006.

FIGURE 2.3 — Polysomnography of Patient in Stage 1 Sleep

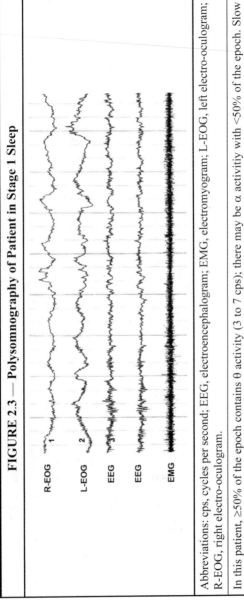

Abbreviations: cps, cycles per second; EEG, electroencephalogram; EMG, electromyogram; L-EOG, left electro-oculogram; R-EOG, right electro-oculogram.

In this patient, ≥50% of the epoch contains θ activity (3 to 7 cps); there may be α activity with <50% of the epoch. Slow rolling eye movements are seen in the EOG channels. Relatively high submental EMG muscle tone is evident.

Illustrated Guide to Polysomnography: Normal Sleep, CD-ROM. Available at: http://aasmnet.org/SleepEdSeries.aspx. Accessed December 13, 2006.

FIGURE 2.4 — Polysomnography of Patient in Stage 2 Sleep

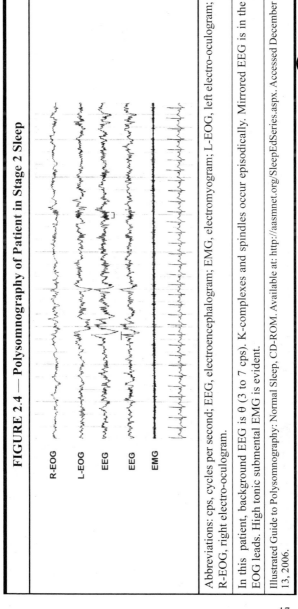

Abbreviations: cps, cycles per second; EEG, electroencephalogram; EMG, electromyogram; L-EOG, left electro-oculogram; R-EOG, right electro-oculogram.

In this patient, background EEG is θ (3 to 7 cps). K-complexes and spindles occur episodically. Mirrored EEG is in the EOG leads. High tonic submental EMG is evident.

Illustrated Guide to Polysomnography: Normal Sleep, CD-ROM. Available at: http://aasmnet.org/SleepEdSeries.aspx. Accessed December 13, 2006.

FIGURE 2.5 — Polysomnography of Patient in Stage 3 Sleep

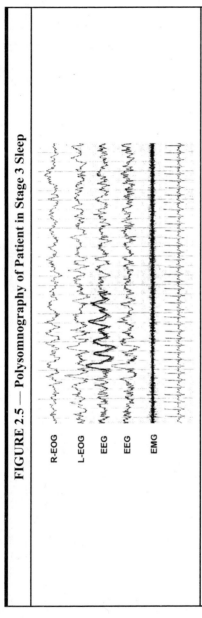

Abbreviations: EEG, electroencephalogram; EMG, electromyogram; L-EOG, left electro-oculogram; R-EOG, right electro-oculogram.

In this patient, >50% of the epoch will have scorable δ activity. EOG channels will mirror δ activity. Submental muscle tone may be slightly reduced.

Illustrated Guide to Polysomnography: Normal Sleep. CD-ROM. Available at: http://aasmnet.org/SleepEdSeries.aspx. Accessed December 13, 2006.

FIGURE 2.6 — Polysomnography of Patient in Stage 4 Sleep

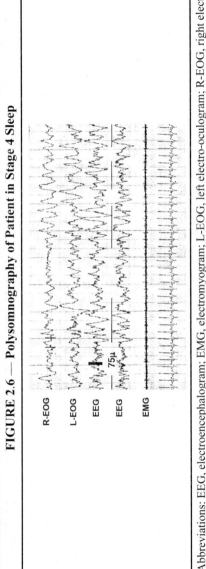

Abbreviations: EEG, electroencephalogram; EMG, electromyogram; L-EOG, left electro-oculogram; R-EOG, right electro-oculogram.

In this patient, >50% of the epoch will have scorable δ EEG activity. The EOG leads will mirror all of the δ EEG activity. Submental EMG activity will be slightly reduced from that of light sleep.

Illustrated Guide to Polysomnography: Normal Sleep, CD-ROM. Available at: http://aasmnet.org/SleepEdSeries.aspx. Accessed December 13, 2006.

FIGURE 2.7 — Polysomnography of Patient in REM Sleep

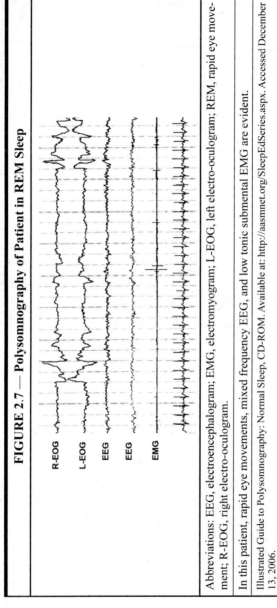

Abbreviations: EEG, electroencephalogram; EMG, electromyogram; L-EOG, left electro-oculogram; REM, rapid eye movement; R-EOG, right electro-oculogram.

In this patient, rapid eye movements, mixed frequency EEG, and low tonic submental EMG are evident.

Illustrated Guide to Polysomnography: Normal Sleep, CD-ROM. Available at: http://aasmnet.org/SleepEdSeries.aspx. Accessed December 13, 2006.

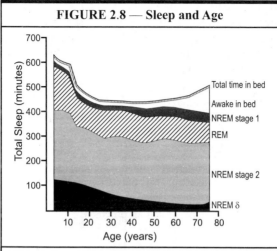

FIGURE 2.8 — Sleep and Age

Total time in bed
Awake in bed
NREM stage 1
REM
NREM stage 2
NREM δ

Total Sleep (minutes)

Age (years)

Abbreviations: NREM, non–rapid eye movement [sleep]; REM, rapid eye movement [sleep].

Erman MK. *J Clin Psychiatry*. 2001;62(suppl 10):9-17.

delta sleep. The loss of delta sleep with age may be a consequence of the diminution in cortical synaptic activity. In contrast, stage 1 sleep increases with age. With aging, there is a general tendency toward sleep fragmentation, characterized by an increase in the frequency of awakenings and brief arousals.

Cognitive mental processes seem to be at a low level during stage 1 sleep since sleepers who are awakened from it usually report experiencing thought fragments or vague images. Most individuals awakened from delta sleep report no mental activity at all. In contrast, most sleepers report dreams when awakened from REM sleep.

Sleep needs are quite variable from individual to individual. Although the average nightly sleep duration is approximately 8 hours, children obtain about 10 hours and the elderly <7 hours. Sleep lengths vary even within similar age groups, with some individuals reportedly requiring as little as 3 hours of nightly sleep. The most prudent answer to the question of "How much sleep do I need?" is that amount of sleep that results in optimal daytime alertness and a sense of mental efficiency and well-being, and in the lack of a tendency to fall asleep unintentionally during the course of the normal daytime hours.

Sleep and wakefulness are believed to be the net effect of the interaction of two opposing processes (**Figure 2.9**):

- Sleep load, which accumulates in proportion to prior wakefulness (homeostatic process)
- Waking signal, whose strength is based on the time of day (circadian process).

Polysomnography is typically performed in specialized facilities called sleep disorders centers and laboratories. In preparation for polysomnography, patients are introduced to their sleeping quarters during their initial office-based evaluation and provisions are

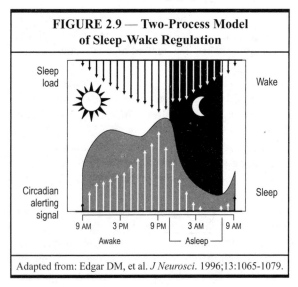

FIGURE 2.9 — Two-Process Model of Sleep-Wake Regulation

Adapted from: Edgar DM, et al. *J Neurosci*. 1996;13:1065-1079.

made for special needs. On the night of the test, they arrive at the laboratory well in advance of the study time to acclimate to the new environment. Studies are conducted in noise-free and private rooms and comfort is maximized by making rooms aesthetically pleasing.

As noted earlier, characterization of sleep stages requires, at the minimum, an EEG, EOG, and EMG of the submentalis. However, a typical clinical polysomnogram also includes monitors for airflow at the nose and mouth, respiratory-effort strain gauges placed around the chest and abdomen, and noninvasive oxygen-saturation monitors that function by introducing a beam of light through the skin. Other parameters include the electrocardiogram and EMG of the anterior tibialis muscles, which are intended to detect periodic leg movements. Finally, a patient's gross body movements are continuously monitored by audiovisual means (**Figure 2.10**).

FIGURE 2.10 — Patient Undergoing Polysomnography

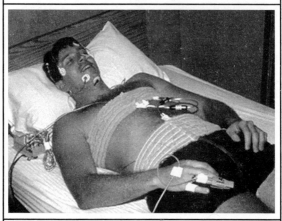

American Academy of Sleep Medicine Slide Set. *Sleep Apnea, Diagnosis, and Treatment*. Westchester, IL: American Academy of Sleep Medicine; 2001.

The most widely recognized accrediting body for sleep disorders centers is the American Academy of Sleep Medicine (www.aasmnet.org). Accredited centers must be staffed by physicians specializing in sleep medicine. Specialty certification in sleep medicine had, for decades, been provided by the independent American Board of Sleep Medicine, an independent board. Beginning in July 2006, however, boards in sleep medicine will be administered exclusively by the American Board of Medical Specialties, in preparation for which physicians must complete training in a 1-year fellowship program that has been approved by the American College of Graduate Medical Education (www.acgme.org). Candidates may enter from one of five disciplines, namely: psychiatry, neurology, pediatrics, internal medicine, and otolaryngology.

REFERENCES

1. National Sleep Foundation. 2003 Sleep in America Poll. WB&A Market Research. Washington, DC.

2. Specchio LM, Prudenzano MP, de Tommaso M, et al. Insomnia, quality of life and psychopathological features. *Brain Res Bull.* 2004;63:385-391.

3. Rechtschaffen A, Bergmann BM, Everson CA, Kushida CA, Gilliland MA. Sleep deprivation in the rat: X. Integration and discussion of the findings. *Sleep.* 1989;12:68-87.

4. Roehrs T. Normal sleep and its variations. In: Kryger MH, Roth T, Dement W, eds. *Principles and Practice of Sleep Medicine.* 4th ed. Philadelphia, Pa: Saunders/Elsevier; 2005:1-23.

3

Insomnia: Definition, Diagnostic Terms, Demographics, and Impairments

Definition

Insomnia is a complaint or a symptom of difficulty with sleep.[1] It is the second most commonly expressed symptom (after pain) in primary care.[2] It is defined as a (repeated) difficulty with[3]:

- Sleep initiation (getting to sleep)
- Sleep duration (waking up too early)
- Sleep consolidation (staying asleep)
- Sleep quality (feeling refreshed).

This sleep difficulty occurs despite adequate time and opportunity for sleep.[3] Many diagnostic systems also stipulate that it must result in daytime impairment for it to be termed insomnia.

Diagnostic Terms and Categorization

Insomnia has been categorized in many different ways over the past 50 years. A commonly utilized method is to classify insomnia according to its duration:

- *Transient insomnia*—also termed acute insomnia[4,5]:
  - Lasts 1 night to a few weeks
  - Can be a result of an acute stressor, such as[6]:
    - Acute medical illness
    - Social stress

- Jet lag
- Change in work shift
- Unfamiliar environment (eg, hotel or hospital bed)
- Drugs (eg, caffeine, alcohol, nicotine, side effect of prescription medications)
  – Typically resolves with relief from the stressor
- *Chronic insomnia*—also termed long-term insomnia[3,4]:
  – Minimum durations differ among various sources, ranging from 1 to 6 months
  – Can wax and wane over time.

This classification system has often been connected with etiologic and management implications, suggesting that acute and transient insomnias are more typically due to adjustment issues that resolve with conservative treatment approaches, whereas the chronic insomnias are due to more serious medical or psychiatric difficulties that require greater investigative effort in order to arrive at the proper diagnosis and treatment. Regrettably, these assumptions have never been substantiated; therefore, this type of categorization may have limited practical value.

The more widely accepted classification scheme, outlined by a recent National Institutes of Health (NIH) State-of-the-Science Conference Statement, categorizes insomnia into primary and comorbid (secondary) types. This is thought to be more useful as it suggests an associated ailment that needs to be identified when insomnia is present (comorbid insomnia). When one is not found, the insomnia is presumed to be a disease in and of itself (primary insomnia). Also, the term "comorbid" was utilized in that conference instead of "secondary" insomnia, suggesting that when insomnia and another major medical or psychiatric disorder coexist, the nature of the connection between the two entities is largely not understood. Insomnia can be caused by the underlying disorder, may be an independent entity, or may conceivably cause the disorder itself. Although the identification of the underlying cause is an important clinical endeavor, this line of thinking paves the road for addressing the insomnia as an independent clinical condition before, during, or after identifying and treating the comorbidity. Primary insomnia is defined more extensively below.

Evidence to substantiate this line of thinking is emerging from various sources, one of which is the research on sleep in depression. Sixty-three percent of individuals with major depression have sleep-related complaints.[4] However, for the first episode of depression, the emergence of insomnia actually precedes the emergence of the depressive episode in 47% of cases; it follows the emergence of the depression 29% of the time. In recurrent depression, insomnia appears first 56% of the time and it follows depression 22% of the time. Although the temporal precedence of insomnia does not imply any causal relationships between insomnia and depression, this highlights the complex relationships that seem to exist between insomnia and its associated disorders.[7]

Figure 3.1 shows the various polysomnographic patterns produced by insomnia. These generally parallel patients' subjective complaints of:

- Difficulty with prolonged sleep latency (difficulty falling asleep)
- Multiple awakenings in the early, middle, or late portions of the night
- Waking up for the day too early.

Many insomniacs are also afflicted with brief arousals, not depicted in the figure, which last <15 seconds. These typically go unrecognized by the sleeper yet may cause the sense of unrefreshing sleep after a full night's sleep.

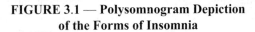

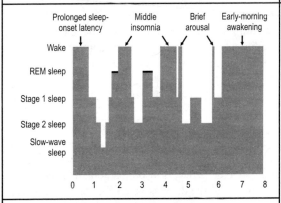

FIGURE 3.1 — Polysomnogram Depiction of the Forms of Insomnia

Abbreviation: REM, rapid eye movement.

McCall V, et al. *J Ambul Monitor*. 1993;6:135-140.

Patients suffering from insomnia typically have a mixture of these patterns. That is, it is quite common for patients who have difficulty falling asleep to also have nocturnal awakenings with difficulty returning to sleep. In **Figure 3.2**, the insomnia symptom most commonly seen is waking up feeling drowsy or tired; close to 75% of all insomniacs report this symptom. Two thirds of these patients wake up in middle of the night, with more than half having trouble falling back to sleep after a middle-of-the-night awakening. Nearly the same number have trouble falling to sleep when they go to bed and, finally, a bit less than half wake up for the day too early.[8]

The forms of the insomnia can change over time—difficulty staying asleep can shift to trouble falling asleep. In one study, symptoms changed in 50% of patients over a 4-month period[9] (**Figure 3.2**). Therefore, physicians must take into account the ever-shifting nature of insomnia when considering treatment options.

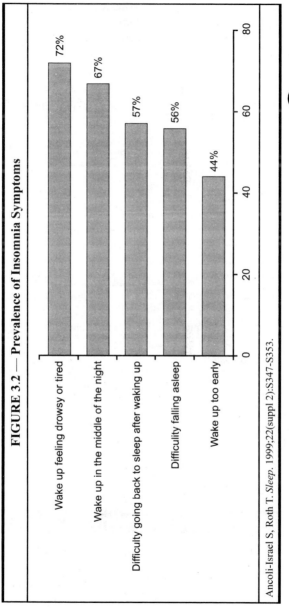

FIGURE 3.2 — Prevalence of Insomnia Symptoms

Wake up feeling drowsy or tired — 72%

Wake up in the middle of the night — 67%

Difficulty going back to sleep after waking up — 57%

Difficulty falling asleep — 56%

Wake up too early — 44%

Ancoli-Israel S, Roth T. *Sleep*. 1999;22(suppl 2):S347-S353.

Primary insomnia is defined as a complaint of insomnia lasting >1 month that:

- Causes clinically significant distress in social or occupational functioning
- Does not occur exclusively during the course of another sleep disorder or mental disorder
- Is not due to a substance or general medical condition.

It is basically an insomnia of no identifiable cause.[3] It is thought to be a state of hyperarousal—a "high idle"—typically beginning in early childhood. Studies have shown that in these patients, there seems to be hypothalamic-pituitary-adrenal axis dysfunction[10] and elevated high-frequency EEG activity during sleep.[11] The prevalence is in debate, but from 10% to 20% of primary insomniacs are diagnosed with these problems.[12] Patients who may present with conditions other than insomnia often state that they have been poor sleepers since childhood. Even though they report next-day consequences, they are not able to nap. They are also more likely to complain of confusion, tension, and depression.[13]

Finally, it should be noted that the great majority of all studies done to determine the efficacy of therapy for insomnia have been in patients with primary insomnia. It is thus in debate whether conclusions drawn and protocols of treatment made for these insomniacs can be extrapolated and applied to insomnia that is comorbid with (and for the most part caused by) another condition.

Demographics

The prevalence of chronic insomnia has been consistent through the past 15 years. Various studies have shown that when insomnia is strictly defined and identified, with medical diagnosis and treatment initiated, chronic insomnia is quite prevalent—around 10% to 20% (**Figure 3.3**).

Over half of American adults report having trouble with sleep a few nights per week or more. The recent NIH State-of-the-Science Conference Statement noted that 30% of the general population has complaints of sleep disruption and 10% has associated symptoms of daytime functional impairment consistent with the diagnosis of insomnia (**Figure 3.4**[14]).

The prevalence of insomnia in primary care clinics is greater. Two studies have shown that >50% of patients who come into a primary care physician's office suffer from a sleep problem.[15,16] One study collected questionnaires from all adult patients coming into the office over a period of time (**Figure 3.5**).[15]

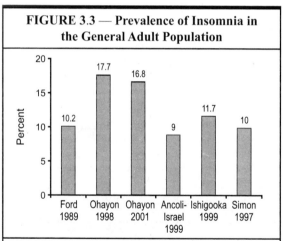

FIGURE 3.3 — Prevalence of Insomnia in the General Adult Population

Insomnia is characterized by sleep disturbance every night for ≥2 weeks or similarly stringent criteria.

Ford DE, Kamerow DB. *JAMA*. 1989;262:1479-1484; Ohayon MM, et al. *Compr Psychiatry*. 1998;39:185-197; Ohayon MM, Roth T. *J Psychosom Res*. 2001;51:745-755; Ancoli-Israel S, Roth T. *Sleep*. 1999;22(suppl 2):S347-S353; Ishigooka J, et al. *Psychiatry Clin Neurosci*. 1999;53:515-522; Simon GE, VonKorff M. *Am J Psychiatry*. 1997;154:1417-1423.

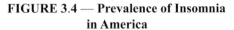

FIGURE 3.4 — Prevalence of Insomnia in America

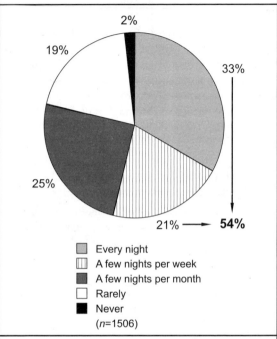

- Every night
- A few nights per week
- A few nights per month
- Rarely
- Never

(*n*=1506)

Forty to 70 million people in the United States have insomnia. 54% of the population reports at least one insomnia symptom a few nights per week.

National Sleep Foundation, 2005. Available at: http://www.sleep foundation.org/_content/hottopics/2005_summary_of_findings. pdf. Accessed December 13, 2006.

The prevalence of insomnia was seen to be 69%, with 50% reporting occasional insomnia and 19% reporting chronic insomnia. As expected, patients with chronic insomnia had the most severe sleep complaints as well as the poorest daytime functioning and exhibited the most help-seeking behaviors. The four factors that predicted that the patient would discuss insomnia with a physician were if the patient:

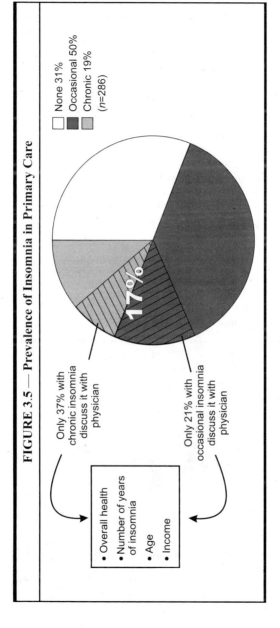

FIGURE 3.5 — Prevalence of Insomnia in Primary Care

None 31%
Occasional 50%
Chronic 19%
(n=286)

17%

Only 37% with chronic insomnia discuss it with physician

Only 21% with occasional insomnia discuss it with physician

- Overall health
- Number of years of insomnia
- Age
- Income

- Was feeling worse physically
- Was afflicted by insomnia for a longer period of time
- Was of an older age
- Had a higher income.

Those who did not bother talking to their doctors about insomnia were typically younger adults without concomitant health problems who had sleep problems for a shorter period of time.

Also quite revealing in this study was the observation that only a fraction (about one third) of insomnia patients mentioned the symptom to their physicians. In a second study, about 50% of primary care patients were found to have insomnia (**Figure 3.6**). But again, only about one third reported the problem spontaneously and only 5% actually sought treatment.[8,15]

Of the patients that come in to see their primary care physicians, the majority of those with insomnia have comorbidities, encompassing 66% to 75% of all insomnia-related sleep complaints.[17] **Figure 3.7**

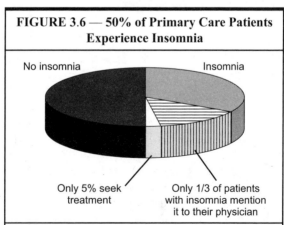

FIGURE 3.6 — 50% of Primary Care Patients Experience Insomnia

No insomnia

Insomnia

Only 5% seek treatment

Only 1/3 of patients with insomnia mention it to their physician

Diagnostic and Statistical Manual of Psychiatric Disorders. 4th ed. Washington, DC: American Psychiatric Association; 2000; Doghramji P. *J Clin Psychiatry.* 2004;65(suppl 16):23-26.

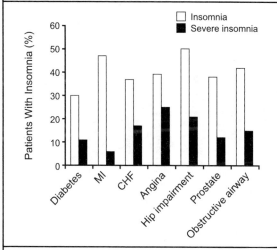

FIGURE 3.7 — Prevalence of Insomnia in Chronic Medical Conditions

Abbreviations: CHF, congestive heart failure; MI, myocardial infarction.

Adapted from: Katz DA, et al. *Arch Intern Med.* 1998;158:1099-1107.

depicts the prevalence of insomnia in various medical conditions. In an Italian study, of the 3284 patients presenting for routine care, 64% had insomnia. In those patients, a wide range of comorbidities were seen, including cardiovascular disease (35%), musculoskeletal disease (28%), gastrointestinal conditions (19%), endocrine conditions (17%), nervous system disease (15%), respiratory conditions (14%), and genitourinary conditions (11%) (**Figure 3.8**).[16] With the exception of respiratory diseases, rates for all of these conditions were slightly higher in individuals with insomnia than in a cohort of 1191 people without insomnia.

Insomnia is also prevalent in psychiatric populations. When we look at all patients with insomnia, around 40% have psychiatric disorders, as depicted in **Figure 3.9**.[18] But if we look at the psychiatric popula-

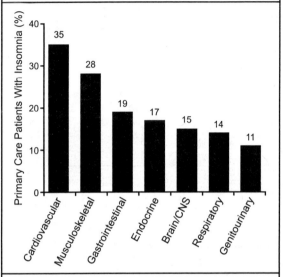

FIGURE 3.8 — Insomnia Comorbidities in Primary Care Patients

Abbreviation: CNS, central nervous system.

Terzano MG, et al. *Sleep Med.* 2004;5:67-75.

tion alone, sleep disturbance is reported by at least 75% of acutely ill psychiatric patients and persists in up to one third of patients even during periods of clinical remission.[19] Moreover, studies of diagnostic patterns in sleep disorders centers have found that the most common primary diagnosis for patients presenting with a complaint of insomnia is a psychiatric illness. In a multicenter study of patients evaluated by clinical interview and polysomnography, 35% of insomniacs had a psychiatric disorder.[20]

In hospitalized patients, who have the greatest severity of comorbidities, insomnia prevalence is also expectedly quite high. In one study of 200 adult patients in a 293-bed general hospital, more than half (56.5%) complained of insomnia. Interestingly,

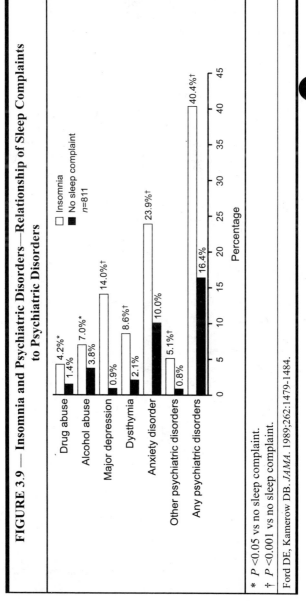

FIGURE 3.9 — Insomnia and Psychiatric Disorders—Relationship of Sleep Complaints to Psychiatric Disorders

Insomnia
No sleep complaint
n=811

Drug abuse — 4.2%* / 1.4%
Alcohol abuse — 7.0%* / 3.8%
Major depression — 14.0%† / 0.9%
Dysthymia — 8.6%† / 2.1%
Anxiety disorder — 23.9%† / 10.0%
Other psychiatric disorders — 5.1%† / 0.8%
Any psychiatric disorders — 40.4%† / 16.4%

Percentage

* P <0.05 vs no sleep complaint.
† P <0.001 vs no sleep complaint.

Ford DE, Kamerow DB. *JAMA.* 1989;262:1479-1484.

insomnia was not mentioned in any of these patients' hospital records, and this symptom predated the hospitalization in many cases. The presence of insomnia was not associated with age, sex, marital status, schooling, or personal income. Half of the 200 patients reported having a history of or a current psychiatric disorder, the most common of which was major depressive disorder (35%). The presence of insomnia had a positive predictive value for major depressive disorder of 46.9%. All the patients with major depressive disorder were symptomatic during the hospitalization. Other psychiatric disorders identified were generalized anxiety disorder (11.5%), panic disorder/agoraphobia (9%), alcohol abuse/dependence (7.5%), psychotic syndrome (5.5%), bipolar disorder (5.5%), social phobia (4%), posttraumatic stress disorder (4%), obsessive-compulsive disorder (4%), dysthymic disorder (2%), and substance abuse/dependence (1%). Only three (1.5%) of the patients in this study had any record of their psychiatric diagnosis in the hospital chart. This showed that hospitalized patients with insomnia have 3.6 times the risk of major depressive disorder; but again, the insomnia as well as the psychiatric disorder often goes unrecognized.[21]

Certain population groups are at higher risk for insomnia (**Table 3.1**). Most obvious are those of rising age. Insomnia is prevalent in elderly patients (>65 years)[22] and, in one study, was seen to exist in close to 60% of the noninstitutionalized elderly.[23] The most common sleep disturbance is sleep discontinuity, where awakenings are noted during the sleep period. Changes in sleep with aging have been reviewed in Chapter 2, *Normal Sleep*.[24] In general, sleep becomes more fragmented and discontinuous. Moreover, seniors are more likely to take naps, suggesting that age-dependent changes reflect a reduced ability to sleep rather than reduced need for sleep.[25] However, these numbers are also greatly due to the elderly's tendency for more infir-

TABLE 3.1 — Risk Factors for Insomnia

Age/Gender	Medical	Psychiatric	Social	Lifestyle	Sleep Environment
• Female • Elderly	• Primary sleep disorder • Obesity • Pain • Arthritis • Alzheimer's • Parkinson's • Heart disease • Respiratory disease • Gastrointestinal disease • Sleep apnea • Restless legs syndrome • Thyroid disorder • Menopause • Testosterone deficiency	• Depression • Anxiety • Tension • Substance or alcohol abuse • Mania or hypomania • Stress • Worry • Conditioning	• Marital separation • Divorce • Death of spouse • Unemployment • Poor working conditions • Lower social status	• Smoking • Drinking alcohol or drinks containing caffeine in the afternoon or evening • Exercising close to bedtime • Irregular schedule • Night-shift work	• Temperature • Lighting • Noise • Interruptions • Partner's sleep habits

Buscemi N et al. Rockville, Md: Agency for Healthcare Research and Quality; June, 2005. AHRQ publication 05-E021-2. Evidence Report/Technology Assessment No. 125; Doghramji PP. *J Clin Psychiatry*. 2001;62(suppl 10):8-26; Doghramji PP. *J Clin Psychiatry*. 2004;65(suppl 16):23-26.

mity, inactivity, dissatisfaction with social life, poor sleep habits,[26] and inappropriate treatment initiated by the patient, family members, physicians, or other care providers[27] (**Figure 3.10**[28]). Finally, recalcitrant insomnia that occurs in dementia is a common cause for institutionalizing the elderly.[26]

Women are at greater risk for insomnia. In one study, women were greater than one and a half times more likely to have insomnia than men.[29] Further, the prevalence of insomnia rises sharply by approximately 40% during the period of transition to menopause and after menopause.[30] Even though sleep quality obviously diminishes during menopause, the pathophysiology involved is yet to be clarified.

Three contributing factors to the development of insomnia in women have been cited. First are the alterations in hormone levels. In fact, the hormonal changes that occur during the various phases of a woman's life (eg, menstruation, pregnancy, and menopause) likely contribute to the high prevalence of sleep problems in all three of those situations.[30] The effect of hot flashes

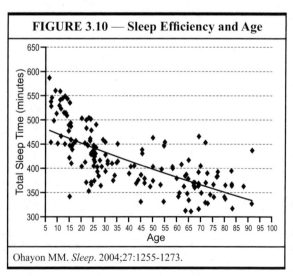

FIGURE 3.10 — Sleep Efficiency and Age

Ohayon MM. *Sleep*. 2004;27:1255-1273.

commonly seen in menopause is controversial. One study reported an association between hot flashes and awakenings from sleep.[31] However, another found no relationship between hot flashes and objective sleep measures of sleep quality.[32] Nevertheless, hot flashes appear to be associated with poor subjective sleep quality.[30] Second, psychiatric problems occur more frequently during menopause and, as clarified earlier, these conditions are more likely to be associated with insomnia. Third, sleep disorders seem to occur more commonly during menopause. As an example, there is more sleep-disordered breathing in postmenopausal women and recent data showed that menopause was an independent risk factor for sleep apnea syndrome.[33]

Other risk factors for insomnia include irregular sleep/wake patterns, as seen in shift workers, whose numbers are increasingly growing in our now 24/7 society. Statistics over the past few years have shown that 15% of full-time wage and salary workers usually work an alternative shift (night, evening, rotating, or on-call shifts).[34] Studies show that 25% of shift workers have insomnia severe enough to meet the diagnosis of shift-work sleep disorder.[35] Finally, additional risk factors include less education, unemployment, separation or divorce, and medical illness.[36]

As a final note regarding epidemiology, insomnia seems to be resilient. Once it develops, insomnia seems to not resolve readily. Among patients with severe symptoms, approximately 80% continue with these for at least a year and 40% continue with symptoms for >5 years.[37] Further, only 56% of insomniacs show remission after 10 years of insomnia.[38]

Consequences of Insomnia

In a study done by Zammit and associates, it was found that those with insomnia had significant impairment in the quality of life (**Figure 3.11**).[39] Moreover,

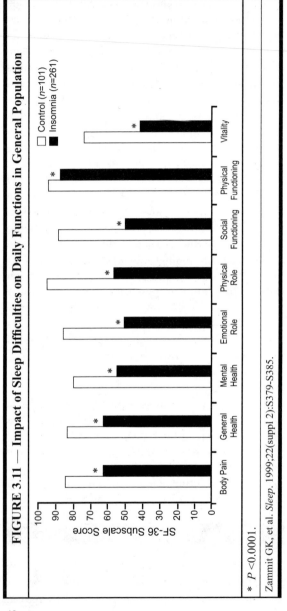

FIGURE 3.11 — Impact of Sleep Difficulties on Daily Functions in General Population

Control (*n*=101)
Insomnia (*n*=261)

SF-36 Subscale Score

Body Pain, General Health, Mental Health, Emotional Role, Physical Role, Social Functioning, Physical Functioning, Vitality

* *P* <0.0001.

Zammit GK, et al. *Sleep*. 1999;22(suppl 2):S379-S385.

these difficulties worsened proportionally with increasing frequency of insomnia. Those with insomnia have also been seen to be at greater risk for developing psychiatric disorders. In a study by Breslau and colleagues, >1000 patients, ages 21 to 30 years, were followed over 3 years. In the patients with no psychiatric problems at the beginning of the study, those who started with insomnia had a substantially greater incidence of new major depression, anxiety disorders, substance abuse disorders, and nicotine dependence by the end of the study (**Figure 3.12**).[40]

Insomnia is associated with an increased risk for injuries and accidents. Those with insomnia have been shown to have 3.5 to 4.5 times more accidents in general, 1.5 times more work-related accidents, and 2.5 times more motor vehicle accidents.[41] Poor sleep quality is a major factor in predicting auto crashes that result from falling asleep at the wheel[42] (**Figure 3.13**[43]).

With these consequences come increases in health care costs and services. In Bavaria, one study showed that those with moderate to severe insomnia saw their physicians 2.5 times more often than their normal-sleeping counterparts.[44] Moreover, those with moderate to severe insomnia were admitted to the hospital nearly twice as often as those without insomnia.[44]

Finally, those with insomnia have been shown to have poorer job performance. A questionnaire by Leger and associates at Stanford University compared the socio-professional and medical consequences of insomniacs and good sleepers.[45] Severe insomniacs reported a higher rate of absenteeism and missed work twice as often as good sleepers. In addition, severe insomniacs had more problems at work than good sleepers, including decreased concentration, difficulty performing tasks, and more work-related accidents.[45]

Insomnia can have unique consequences in the elderly population. Those >65 years of age with insomnia suffer from a greater number of falls than their

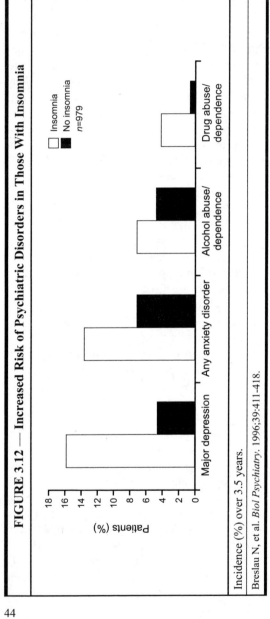

FIGURE 3.12 — Increased Risk of Psychiatric Disorders in Those With Insomnia

Incidence (%) over 3.5 years.

Breslau N, et al. *Biol Psychiatry.* 1996;39:411-418.

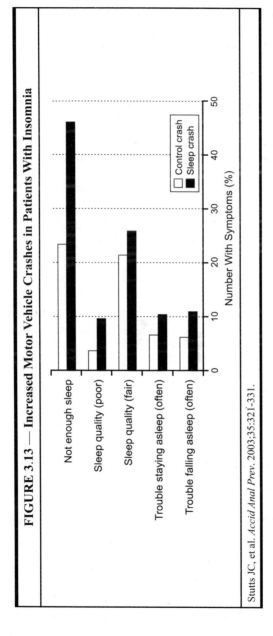

FIGURE 3.13 — Increased Motor Vehicle Crashes in Patients With Insomnia

Stutts JC, et al. *Accid Anal Prev.* 2003;35:321-331.

counterparts without insomnia. In one study of >34,000 nursing home patients, those with insomnia were seen to fall 1.52 times more often than those without insomnia. This number was not attributable to hypnotic use, and use of these medications was not predictive of fall. In fact, those with insomnia who were treated had less falls (1.32 times compared with 1.52).[46]

REFERENCES

1. *Diagnostic and Statistical Manual of Mental Disorders*. 4th ed. Washington, DC: American Psychiatric Association; 2000.

2. Moldofsky H. Pain and insomnia: what every clinician should know. Available at: http://www.medscape.com/view-article/494872. Accessed December 13, 2006.

3. National Institutes of Health. National Institutes of Health State of the Science Conference Statement on Manifestations and Management of Chronic Insomnia in Adults; June 13-15, 2005. *Sleep*. 2005;28:1049-1057.

4. Doghramji K. Treatment strategies for sleep disturbance in patients with depression. *J Clin Psychiatry*. 2003;64(suppl 14):24-29.

5. Czeisler CA, Winkelman JW, Richardson GS. Sleep disorders. In: Kasper DL, Braunwald E, Fauci AS, Hauser SL, Longo DL, Jameson JL, eds. *Harrison's Principles of Internal Medicine*. 16th ed. New York, NY: McGraw-Hill Companies; 2005.

6. Lippmann S, Mazour I, Shahab H. Insomnia: therapeutic approach. *South Med J*. 2001;94:866-873.

7. Ohayon MM, Roth T. Place of chronic insomnia in the course of depressive and anxiety disorders. *J Psychiatr Res*. 2003;37:9-15.

8. Ancoli-Israel S, Roth T. Characteristics of insomnia in the United States: results of the 1991 National Sleep Foundation Survey. I. *Sleep*. 1999;22(suppl 2):S347-S353.

9.   Hohagen F, Rink K, Kappler C, et al. Prevalence and treatment of insomnia in general practice. A longitudinal study. *Eur Arch Psychiatry Clin Neurosci*. 1993;242:329-336.

10. Richardson GS, Roth T. Future directions in the management of insomnia. *J Clin Psychiatry*. 2001;62(suppl 10):39-45.

11. Perlis ML, Kehr EL, Smith MT, Andrews PJ, Orff H, Giles DE. Temporal and stagewise distribution of high frequency EEG activity in patients with primary and secondary insomnia and in good sleeper controls. *J Sleep Res*. 2001;10:93-104.

12. Ohayon MM, Caulet M, Lemoine P. Cormorbidity of mental and insomnia disorders in the general population. *Comp Psychiatry*. 1998;39:185-197.

13. Bonnet MH, Arand DL. The consequences of a week of insomnia. *Sleep*. 1996;19:453-461.

14. National Sleep Foundation. 2005. Available at: http://www.sleepfoundation.org/_content/hottopics/2005_summary_of_findings.pdf. Accessed December 13, 2006.

15. Shochat T, Umphress J, Israel AG, Ancoli-Israel S. Insomnia in primary care patients. *Sleep*. 1999;22(suppl 2):S359-S365.

16. Terzano MG, Parrino L, Cirignotta F, et al. Studio Morfeo: insomnia in primary care, a survey conducted on the Italian population. *Sleep Med*. 2004;5:67-75.

17. Ohayon MM, Partinen M. Insomnia and global sleep dissatisfaction in Finland. *J Sleep Res*. 2002;11:339-346.

18. Ford DE, Kamerow DB. Epidemiologic study of sleep disturbances and psychiatric disorders. An opportunity for prevention? *JAMA*. 1989;262:1479-1484.

19. Sweetwood H, Grant I, Kripke DF, Gerst MS, Yager J. Sleep disorder over time: psychiatric correlates among males. *Br J Psychiatry*. 1980;136:456-462.

20. Coleman RM, Roffwarg HP, Kennedy SJ, et al. Sleep-wake disorders based on a polysomnographic diagnosis. A national cooperative study. *JAMA*. 1982;247:997-1003.

21. Rocha FL, Hara C, Rodrigues CV, et al. Is insomnia a marker for psychiatric disorders in general hospitals? *Sleep Med.* 2005;6:549-553.

22. Foley DJ, Monjan AA, Brown SL, Simonsick EM, Wallace RB, Blazer DG. Sleep complaints among elderly persons: an epidemiologic study of three communities. *Sleep.* 1995;18:425-432.

23. McCall WV. Sleep in the elderly: burden, diagnosis, and treatment. *Prim Care Companion J Clin Psychiatry.* 2004;6:9-20.

24. Roth T, Roehrs T. Sleep organization and regulation. *Neurology.* 2000;54(suppl 1):S2-S7.

25. Richardson G, Doghramji K. Insomnia: Specialist's Edition. *Clinical Symposia.* 2005;55:1-39.

26. Foley D, Ancoli-Israel S, Britz P, Walsh J. Sleep disturbances and chronic disease in older adults: results of the 2003 National Sleep Foundation Sleep in America Survey. *J Psychosom Res.* 2004;56:497-502.

27. Neubauer DN. Sleep problems in the elderly. *Am Fam Physician.* 1999;59:2551-2560.

28. Ohayon MM, Carskadon MA, Guilleminault C, Vitiello MV. Meta-analysis of quantitative sleep parameters from childhood to old age in healthy individuals: developing normative sleep values across the human lifespan. *Sleep.* 2004;27:1255-1273.

29. Li RH, Wing YK, Ho SC, Fong SY. Gender differences in insomnia—a study in the Hong Kong Chinese population. *J Psychosom Res.* 2002;53:601-609.

30. Zee PC. Expert column—Insomnia and Menopause. 2004. Available at: http://www.medscape.com/viewarticle/484767?src=search. Accessed December 13, 2006.

31. Woodward S, Freedman RR. The thermoregulatory effects of menopausal hot flashes on sleep. *Sleep.* 1994;17:497-501.

32. Polo-Kantola P, Erkkola R, Irjala K, Helenius H, Pullinen S, Polo O. Climacteric symptoms and sleep quality. *Obstet Gynecol.* 1999;94:219-224.

33. Moline ML, Broch L, Zak R. Sleep in women across the life cycle from adulthood through menopause. *Med Clin North Am*. 2004;88:705-736.

34. Bureau of Labor Statistics. Workers on Flexible and Shift Schedules 2004 Summary. Available at: http://www.bls.gov/news.release/flex.nr0.htm. Accessed December 13, 2006.

35. Ohayon MM, Lemoine P, Arnaud-Briant V, Dreyfus M. Prevalence and consequences of sleep disorders in a shift worker population. *J Psychosom Res*. 2002;53:577-583.

36. Sateia MJ, Doghramji K, Hauri PJ, Morin CM. Evaluation of chronic insomnia. An American Academy of Sleep Medicine review. *Sleep*. 2000;23:243-308.

37. Hohagen F, Kappler C, Schramm E, et al. Prevalence of insomnia in elderly general practice attenders and the current treatment modalities. *Acta Psychiatr Scand*. 1994;90:102-108.

38. Janson C, Lindberg E, Gislason T, Elmasry A, Boman G. Insomnia in men—a 10-year prospective population based study. *Sleep*. 2001;24:425-430.

39. Zammit GK, Weiner J, Damato N, Sillup GP, McMillan CA. Quality of life in people with insomnia. *Sleep*. 1999;22(suppl 2):S379-S385.

40. Breslau N, Roth T, Rosenthal L, Andreski P. Sleep disturbance and psychiatric disorders: a longitudinal epidemiological study of young adults. *Biol Psychiatry*. 1996;39:411-418.

41. Stoller MK. Economic effects of insomnia. *Clin Ther*. 1994;16:873-897; discussion 854.

42. Sabbagh-Ehrlich S, Friedman L, Richter ED. Working conditions and fatigue in professional truck drivers at Israeli ports. *Injury Prevention*. 2005;11:110-114.

43. Stutts JC, Wilkins JW, Scott Osberg J, Vaughn BV. Driver risk factors for sleep-related crashes. *Accid Anal Prev*. 2003;35:321-331.

44. Weyerer S, Dilling H. Prevalence and treatment of insomnia in the community: results from the Upper Bavarian Field Study. *Sleep*. 1991;14:392-398.

45. Leger D, Guilleminault C, Bader G, Levy E, Paillard M. Medical and socio-professional impact of insomnia. *Sleep*. 2002;25:625-629.

46. Avidan AY, Fries BE, James ML, Szafara KL, Wright GT, Chervin RD. Insomnia and hypnotic use, recorded in the minimum data set, as predictors of falls and hip fractures in Michigan nursing homes. *J Am Geriatr Soc*. 2005;53:955-962.

4 Differential Diagnosis

Primary Insomnia

The *Diagnostic and Statistical Manual of Mental Disorders* (DSM-IV-TR) organizes sleep disorders into four major categories according to presumed causes[1]:

- Primary insomnia (essentially insomnia with no identifiable cause)
- Related to another mental disorder
- Due to a general medical condition
- Substance induced.

The latter three obviously have causes or comorbidities and, by definition, the first is a sleep problem with no identifiable cause. The DSM-IV-TR identifies the essential features of primary insomnia as follows:

- The predominant symptom is difficulty initiating or maintaining sleep or nonrestorative sleep for at least 1 month.
- The sleep disturbance (or associated daytime fatigue) causes clinically significant distress or impairment in social, occupational, or other important areas of functioning.
- The sleep disturbance does not occur exclusively during the course of narcolepsy, breathing-related sleep disorder, circadian rhythm sleep disorder, or parasomnia.
- The disturbance does not occur exclusively during the course of another mental disorder (eg, major depressive disorder, generalized anxiety disorder, delirium).
- The disturbance is not due to the direct physiologic effects of a substance (eg, drug abuse, medication) or a general medical condition.

As already described in Chapter 3, *Insomnia: Definition, Diagnostic Terms, Demographics, and Impairments*, consensus is emerging regarding the notion of primary insomnia, sometimes referred to as the "insomnia syndrome," as an independent disorder that does not have any identifiable cause. The International Classification of Sleep Disorders[2] does not recognize a category of primary insomnia but discusses the following three free-standing insomnia conditions that can be subsumed within the rubric of primary insomnia:

- *Psychophysiologic insomnia:* A disorder of somatized tension and learned sleep-preventing associations that result in a complaint of insomnia and associated decreased functioning during wakefulness
- *Idiopathic insomnia:* Lifelong inability to obtain adequate sleep that is presumably due to an abnormality of the neurologic control of the sleep-wake system
- *Sleep-state misperception:* A disorder in which a complaint of insomnia occurs without objective evidence of sleep disturbance, or in which the subjective complaint far outweighs the objective evidence for it.

Primary insomnia is thought to occur in 1% to 2% of the population[3] and to represent 25% of all insomnias.[4]

Patients with primary insomnia sleep less at night yet they do not exhibit evidence of sleepiness during daytime sleep laboratory tests.[5,6] The etiology of the disorder is poorly understood. As mentioned in Chapter 3, numerous physiologic correlates have been identified in this disorder. Many believe that it is a learned behavior that can be unlearned, yet others consider it a distinct physiologic disorder, possibly with hereditary components. Evidence to support this understanding is derived from studies demonstrating increased basal metabolic rates, increased electroencephalogram (EEG) frequency patterns during sleep, increased multiple sleep latency scores, cognitive hyperarousal ("I can't shut off my mind at night"), and increased glucose metabolism during sleep on functional neuroimaging studies. Metabolic rates as measured by oxygen consumption are also significantly elevated in these insomniacs. One study demonstrated this by using caffeine to create a state of arousal in normal subjects. They not only developed insomnia as expected, but also had an increased metabolic state and complained, as do insomniacs, that their vigor was significantly lower with caffeine.[7]

Primary insomnia patients have also been seen to exhibit increased sympathetic nervous system activity, elevated core body temperature, and elevated levels of circulating catecholamines. The degree of cortisol elevation is related to the severity of the insomnia.[8] Overactivity of the hypothalamic-pituitary-adrenal axis is also noted, as evidenced by elevated cortisol levels and lower levels of growth hormone during sleep.[9]

As noted above, primary insomnia can also be seen as the product of learned associations that are superimposed upon a vulnerable neurophysiologic system. An individual who is predisposed to insomnia, possibly through a hereditary tendency, can easily develop the condition following exposure to stressors in later life. As the stressor abates, the insomnia does not abate since it is now fueled by learned, maladaptive behaviors and cognitions (**Figure 4.1**).[10]

Some individuals who complain of insomnia are actually short sleepers. They represent individuals who have a relatively diminished need for sleep, as they sleep less than the population mean of 8 hours yet do not exhibit evidence of daytime impairment. They are typically energetic, active, and derive pleasure from their work, which many see as a natural consequence of having more waking hours to fill. Both Thomas Edison and Napoleon Bonaparte are purported to have been

FIGURE 4.1 — Factors in the Genesis and Progression of Primary Insomnia

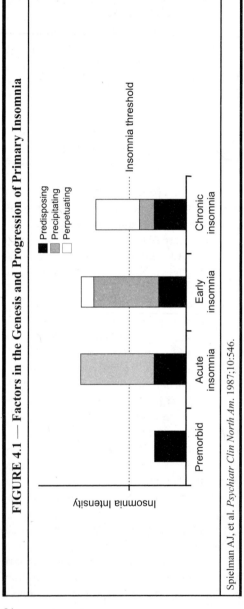

Spielman AJ, et al. *Psychiatr Clin North Am.* 1987;10:546.

successful "short sleepers."[11] The clinical approach to short sleepers involves reassurance that the short sleep hours do not represent a clinical condition plus education regarding sleep needs. On the flip side, some people naturally sleep longer, 9 hours or more. They tend to display a devout nonconformist personality and have been found to be more likely to question and complain about politics and economic situations. Albert Einstein may have been a classic "long sleeper."[11]

Comorbid (Secondary) Insomnia

As discussed in Chapter 3, comorbid insomnias are more commonly encountered than primary insomnia. In the workup of insomnia, it is most common that the primary care physician finds a comorbidity with the insomnia. The term "comorbidity" has replaced the term "secondary" by the National Institutes of Health recent conference, as the report states:

"Most cases of insomnia are comorbid with other conditions. Historically, this has been termed 'secondary insomnia.' However, the limited understanding of mechanistic pathways in chronic insomnia precludes drawing firm conclusions about the nature of these associations or direction of causality. Furthermore, there is concern that the term secondary insomnia may promote undertreatment. Therefore, we propose that the term 'comorbid insomnia' may be more appropriate."[12]

Some of these conditions are noted in **Table 4.1**.[13]

Psychiatric Comorbidity

Most of the comorbidities associated with insomnia are psychiatric in nature (**Figure 4.2**).[14] Therefore, the clinician who evaluates insomnia should have a

TABLE 4.1 — Common Psychiatric and Medical Causes of Insomnia

Psychiatric Causes
- Mood disorders (depression, bipolar disorder, dysthymia)
- Anxiety disorders (generalized anxiety disorder, panic disorder, posttraumatic stress disorder)
- Substance abuse
- Life stressors
- Conditioning (associating the bed with wakefulness)
- Mania or hypomania
- Dementia
- Eating disorders
- Schizophrenia

Primary Sleep Disorders
- Obstructive sleep apnea
- Restless legs syndrome
- Periodic limb movement disorder
- Circadian rhythm disorder
- Parasomnias
- Narcolepsy

Medical Causes
- Chronic pain
- Cardiovascular disease (congestive heart failure, angina)
- Drug or alcohol intoxication or withdrawal
- Endocrine disorders (thyroid imbalance, dysfunctional uterine bleeding)
- Menopause
- Rheumatic disease (fibromyalgia, arthritis, ankylosing spondylitis, Sjögren's syndrome)
- Pulmonary disease (chronic obstructive pulmonary disease, asthma, pneumonia)
- Neurologic disorders (Parkinson's disease, Alzheimer's disease, multiple sclerosis, uncontrolled migraines, brain tumor, traumatic brain injury)
- Urologic disease (benign prostatic hyperplasia, overactive bladder)

Continued

- Gastrointestinal disease (gastroesophageal reflux disease, peptic ulcer disease, irritable bowel syndrome)
- Acquired immunodeficiency syndrome (AIDS)
- Chronic fatigue syndrome
- Lyme disease
- Dermatologic disorders (nocturnal pruritus)
- Systemic cancer

Doghramji PP. *Postgraduate Medicine Special Report*. December, 2004:14-22.

high index of suspicion for an underlying psychiatric disorder. Clinical experience suggests that patients who have insomnia as a result of a psychiatric disorder may not appreciate the connection between insomnia and their emotional impairment. They may also not be aware of the psychiatric disorder itself. Therefore, in clinical settings, the stigmata of individual psychiatric conditions should be carefully elicited. As noted in **Figure 4.3**,[15] anxiety disorders are the most frequent psychiatric diagnoses in patients with insomnia.

Insomnia confers a heightened risk for the presence of a psychiatric disorder. It is no surprise that when most primary care providers see insomnia, they first consider the possibility of a coexisting psychiatric disorder (**Figure 4.3**).[15] Nevertheless, the relationship between insomnia and psychiatric disorders is somewhat complex. As discussed in Chapter 3, it is more common for insomnia to emerge prior to rather than during or following certain psychiatric disorders, such as depression.[16] In fact, insomnia often is predictive of the future emergence of a psychiatric disorder. When patients experiencing insomnia were followed for 3.5 years, Breslau and colleagues[17] found that they had a significantly higher rate of development of new psychiatric disorders over that period of time (**Figure 4.4**). In the Johns Hopkins Precursors Study, which involved an even longer follow-up period, >1000 medical students were followed over 40 years; medical

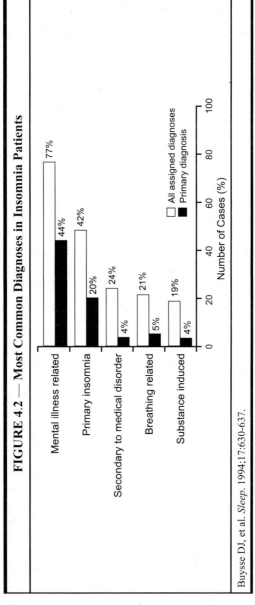

FIGURE 4.2 — Most Common Diagnoses in Insomnia Patients

Mental illness related — 77% (All assigned diagnoses), 44% (Primary diagnosis)

Primary insomnia — 42% (All assigned diagnoses), 20% (Primary diagnosis)

Secondary to medical disorder — 24% (All assigned diagnoses), 4% (Primary diagnosis)

Breathing related — 21% (All assigned diagnoses), 5% (Primary diagnosis)

Substance induced — 19% (All assigned diagnoses), 4% (Primary diagnosis)

Number of Cases (%)

□ All assigned diagnoses
■ Primary diagnosis

Buysse DJ, et al. *Sleep*. 1994;17:630-637.

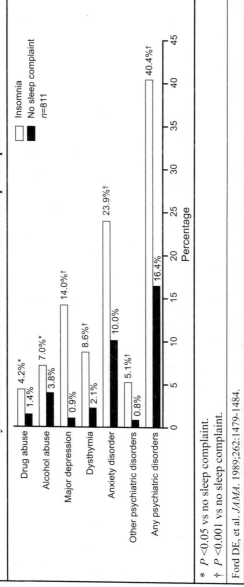

FIGURE 4.3 — Significantly More Respondents With Insomnia Had One or More Psychiatric Disorders vs Those With No Sleep Complaints

Legend:
- Insomnia
- No sleep complaint
- n=811

Category	Insomnia	No sleep complaint
Drug abuse	4.2%*	1.4%
Alcohol abuse	7.0%*	3.8%
Major depression	14.0%†	0.9%
Dysthymia	8.6%†	2.1%
Anxiety disorder	23.9%†	10.0%
Other psychiatric disorders	5.1%†	0.8%
Any psychiatric disorders	40.4%†	16.4%

Percentage

* P <0.05 vs no sleep complaint.
† P <0.001 vs no sleep complaint.

Ford DE, et al. *JAMA.* 1989;262:1479-1484.

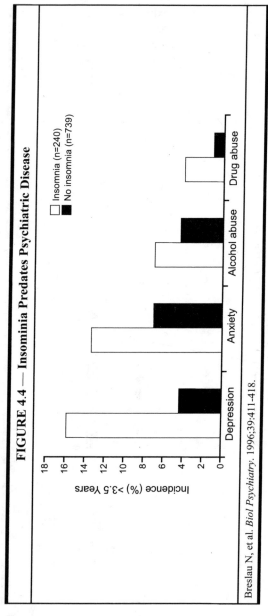

FIGURE 4.4 — Insominia Predates Psychiatric Disease

Incidence (%) >3.5 Years

Depression   Anxiety   Alcohol abuse   Drug abuse

☐ Insomnia (n=240)
■ No insomnia (n=739)

Breslau N, et al. *Biol Psychiatry*. 1996;39:411-418.

students who complained of insomnia during medical school but who did not exhibit evidence of comorbidity were at greater risk for developing depression over the ensuing 40 years (**Figure 4.5**).[18] It is striking that depression did not begin to occur until 17 years after the development of the insomnia. Although such data do not confirm a causal relationship between insomnia and psychiatric conditions, they suggest a bidirectional relationship between the two. They also suggest that in clinical settings, the presence of insomnia should alert clinicians to the possibility of an impending psychiatric condition.

The presence of a psychiatric disorder also confers a heightened risk for insomnia. Eighty percent of depressed patients complain of sleep-related disturbances, including:

- Difficulty in falling asleep
- Difficulty in staying asleep
- Early morning awakening.

FIGURE 4.5 — Cumulative Incidence of Depression in Insomnia

Insomnia	Total	Cases
Yes	137	23
No	887	76

$P = 0.0005$

Insomnia								
Yes	137	135	133	127	117	106	99	27	9
No	887	877	859	838	799	740	616	382	216

Number of men included at each time point.

Chang P, et al. *Am J Epidemiol*. 1997;146:105-114.

Whereas it was once thought that the latter two symptoms were more common in depressed individuals, studies of unmedicated depressed patients suggest that these three symptoms are equally likely to occur in a depressed patient. Therefore, difficulty in falling asleep is as likely to represent a depressive phenomenon as a difficulty in staying asleep.[19]

Insomnia that occurs during a depressive episode should, at least in theory, be mitigated following management of the underlying depression. However, insomnia persists in nearly half of the individuals whose depression has been been successfully managed,[20] in which case it may be either a persistent side effect of the antidepressant or may represent the symptom of a persistent, subsyndromal depression. Persistent insomnia in the depressed patient is important to monitor since it is predictive of the recurrence of the depression at a later date.[21]

The complex relationship that exists between insomnia and various psychiatric disorders as discussed here also exists between insomnia and depression in particular. Sleep problems have been seen to occur before, during, and after the onset of a major depressive episode. In fact, in the case of the first episode of depression, the onset of insomnia precedes depression 47% of the time and follows depression 29% of the time. In the case of recurrent depression, insomnia appears first 56% of the time and follows depression 22% of the time.[16]

Another sobering note is that the presence of insomnia in the depressed patient introduces clinical complications, as it may be predictive of suicidal tendency.[21] In one prospective study of 34 suicides over 10 years among 954 patients with major affective disorder, severe insomnia was one of the main symptoms that differentiated suicides within 1 year from the majority of depressed nonsuicides.[22] Additionally, a study of 100 patients who had attempted suicide and were brought to an emergency room revealed that 92% of patients complained of partial insomnia (global insomnia in 46%).[23] Such data necessitate the raising of one's index of suspicion for the development of a psychiatric disorder in patients presenting with insomnia. What has yet to be shown is whether early intervention and treatment of insomnia that is not comorbid lessens the likelihood of future development of psychiatric disorders.

4

■ Insomnia and Anxiety Disorders

Insomnia and anxiety disorders often coexist. As described, the process of insomnia development involves—at least in the case of primary insomnia—mental and/or physical activation and anxiety at bedtime and/or after falling asleep. It is not surprising, therefore, that 24% of those in the community who experience insomnia have a diagnosable anxiety disorder. Even in insomniacs who do not have a current psychiatric disorder, the persistence of insomnia confers an increased risk for the development of future anxiety disorders.[15] In turn, patients who have anxiety disorders are at high risk for disturbed sleep. The sleep of generalized anxiety-disorder patients is characterized by an increased time required to fall asleep and increased awakenings and arousals after falling asleep, as well as a decrease in the percentage of time slept in deeper stages (3 and 4) of sleep.[24,25] Patients with posttraumatic stress disorder (PTSD) frequently awaken with startle symptoms and physiologic arousal following trauma-related nightmares, typically during rapid eye movement (REM) sleep.[26]

When a patient presents with the primary symptoms of insomnia and anxiety, the first step should be to determine whether the difficulty represents primarily insomnia or an anxiety disorder. In the case of the former, the anxiety is from the anticipation of another sleepless night. These patients' mind races with random thoughts as they become focused upon and brood over their sleeplessness, which, in turn, aggravates their insomnia even further. A situational pattern of insomnia is common, in which a patient will typically have greater difficulty falling asleep in their own bedroom and will be often amazed to find that they fall asleep more easily when away from home. This occurs because their own bedroom triggers the fear of sleeplessness and the cascade of anxiety. In contrast, when the primary difficulty is an anxiety disorder, anxiety is present day and night. In addition, the patient's focus is usually not only on the insomnia itself but also on ancillary aspects of the disorder, such as distressing nightmares in PTSD and compulsions in obsessive-compulsive disorder. Additionally, the situational aspects of primary insomnia are not seen.

■ Insomnia and Bipolar Disorder

During manic episodes, there is decreased need for sleep. On the other hand, bipolar patients who are in the depressed phase of their illness can switch into a manic episode following sleep loss from any reason, including jet lag and work schedules.[27,28] Therefore, insomnia is an important symptom to follow clinically in the bipolar patient. [29]

■ Insomnia and Schizophrenia

In schizophrenia, insomnia is a common symptom, although it is seldom the predominant complaint. It occurs regardless of either medication status (never medicated or presently on medications) or the phase of the clinical course (acute or chronic). Patients typically have both sleep-onset and sleep-maintenance insomnia. Patients often complain of daytime sleepiness, but it is unclear whether this is due to the distorted sleep architecture or to the disease itself or a combination of both.[30]

■ Insomnia and Attention-Deficit Hyperactivity Disorder (ADHD)

Sleep difficulties are reportedly present in between 25% and 50% of children with ADHD, compared with 7% of normal controls.[31] The etiology of disturbed sleep in ADHD is poorly understood. In adults, it may be secondary to other comorbid psychiatric disorders, such as major depressive disorder, anxiety disorders, personality disorders, substance abuse disorders, or bipolar disorder.[32] However, in one study of adults with ADHD and no identifiable psychiatric comorbidity, sleep was still impaired. Polysomnography showed increased nocturnal motor activity, and the degree of objective sleep disturbance was disproportionately higher than that reported on subjective measures.[33]

The increased nocturnal motor activity of ADHD patients may be related to restless legs syndrome (RLS) in ADHD adults. One study did in fact demonstrate that patients diagnosed with RLS had symptoms compatible with ADHD. The authors speculated that RLS could manifest as hyperactivity and, by producing poor sleep quality, could lead to cognitive impairment, including lack of concentration. An alternative hypothesis is that RLS and ADHD may be part of a single symptom complex related to dopaminergic dysfunction.[34] However, even though this and other data show an association between ADHD and RLS, further clinical trials and epidemiologic studies are needed to quantify the relationship and the degree of association.[35] Nonetheless, the clinician who sees either condition should address the possibility of coexistence of the two.

■ Insomnia and Substance Abuse

The association between insomnia and substance abuse is high (**Table 4.1**, **Figure 4.2**, and **Figure 4.3**). Studies consistently show that use of illicit drugs can lead to insomnia and also that those with insomnia have a greater likelihood of abusing drugs. The clinician should keenly be aware of this bidirectional relationship and address each condition accordingly.

Medical Comorbidity

Medical conditions are associated with insomnia (**Table 4.1** and **Figure 4.6**). In a survey of >3000 patients presenting to a primary care clinic, the majority (64%) had insomnia and a wide range of comorbid conditions. Compared with a cohort of 1191 patients without insomnia, higher rates of all medical conditions were found in insomnia patients (cardiovascular, musculoskeletal, gastrointestinal, endocrine, central nervous system, and genitourinary disease) with the exception of respiratory disease. In another, longitudinal study, patients with chronic medical conditions and insomnia were followed over 2 years. Sixteen percent had severe insomnia and 34% had mild insomnia at baseline. At 2-year follow-up, 59% of patients with mild insomnia and 83% of patients with severe insomnia at baseline still had sleep problems, indicating the resiliency of insomnia in chronic medical conditions (**Table 4.2**). This provides the foundation for clinicians to address medical conditions that disturb sleep when addressing insomnia, especially cardiopulmonary disease, painful musculoskeletal conditions, and prostate problems.[36]

In a variety of conditions, awakenings during sleep may be protective. For example, in gastroesophageal reflux disease, esophageal acid clearance during sleep is enhanced by the arousal response; in chronic obstructive pulmonary disease, the awakening process restores SaO_2 levels.[37] Therefore, symptomatic management of insomnia in such individuals risks the possibility of an exacerbation of the underlying disease process. These data emphasize the need to perform a thorough medical evaluation in patients presenting with insomnia.

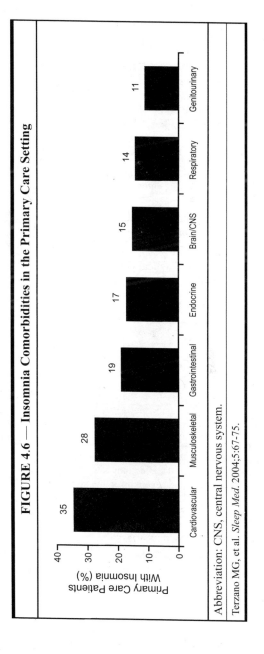

FIGURE 4.6 — Insomnia Comorbidities in the Primary Care Setting

Abbreviation: CNS, central nervous system.

Terzano MG, et al. *Sleep Med.* 2004;5:67-75.

TABLE 4.2 — Clinical Risk Factors Associated With Mild and Severe Insomnia at Baseline*

	Mild Insomnia	Severe Insomnia
Physician-Diagnosed Conditions		
Major depression	2.6[†]	8.2[†]
Subthreshold depression	2.2[†]	3.4[†]
Myocardial infarction	1.9[‡]	0.9
Congestive heart failure	1.6[§]	2.5[†]
Diabetes mellitus	0.8	1.0
Patient-Reported Comorbidities		
Angina pectoris	1.3[§]	1.3
Obstructive airway disease	1.6[‡]	1.5[§]
Back problems	1.4[†]	1.5[‡]
Hip impairment	2.2[‡]	2.7[‡]
Osteoarthritis	1.4[§]	1.6
Rheumatoid arthritis	1.0	1.3
Peptic ulcer	0.9	1.8[§]
Bowel problems	0.9	0.9
Prostate problems	1.6[‡]	1.4
Urinary tract infection	1.1	1.0

* Values are odds ratios adjusted for sociodemographic variables, health habits, and study site. The dependent variables are mild and severe insomnia at baseline.
† $P \leq 0.001$.
‡ $P \leq 0.01$.
§ $P \leq 0.05$.

Katz DA, et al. *Arch Intern Med.* 1998;158:1099-1107.

■ Insomnia and Aging

The increased prevalence of insomnia in the elderly may be related to a direct effect of the aging process on the mechanisms that control sleep and wakefulness, or it may be a product of the medical and psychiatric conditions that increase in prevalence with age. In a poll taken by the National Sleep Foundation,[38] aging men and women reported that waking up to go to the bathroom was by far the most prevalent of the medical symptoms that disturbed sleep. Interestingly, despite one intuiting that prostate problems in men would cause them to have more disturbed sleep, prevalence of waking to go to the bathroom was higher among women (**Figure 4.7**). With more and more studies showing that sleep disruption, especially in the elderly, leads to more morbidity and mortality, especially via cerebrovascular and cardiovascular disease,[39] the clinician may extrapolate (until definitive studies either confirm or deny) that identifying and treating nocturia may be more than just treating a nuisance problem.

■ Insomnia and Menopause

Insomnia is more prevalent among women than men throughout the entire life span but especially so during the period of transition that is menopause. Following the onset of menopause, the prevalence of insomnia rises, with as many as 61% of postmenopausal women reporting insomnia symptoms.[40] Factors that may contribute to insomnia during menopause include hot flashes, hormonal changes, sleep disorders (primary insomnia, RLS, obstructive sleep apnea), and psychiatric disorders. The general approach to treating these patients includes good sleep hygiene (as part of or separate from cognitive behavioral therapy) and medications. Hormone replacement therapy (HRT) during menopause has not been clearly shown to help insomnia, as results from trials have varied depending on the specific type of hormone or hormone combina-

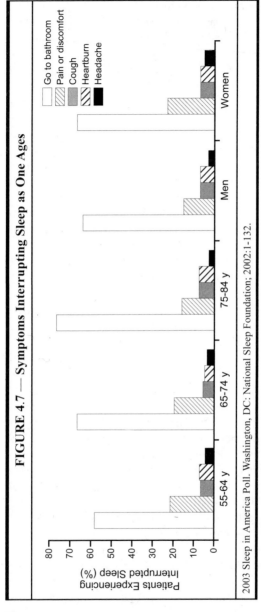

FIGURE 4.7 — Symptoms Interrupting Sleep as One Ages

Go to bathroom
Pain or discomfort
Cough
Heartburn
Headache

Patients Experiencing Interrupted Sleep (%)

55-64 y   65-74 y   75-84 y   Men   Women

2003 Sleep in America Poll. Washington, DC: National Sleep Foundation; 2002:1-132.

tion used. Therefore, there is no consensus regarding the role of HRT for menopausal sleep disruption[41] (see Chapter 7, *Management: General Considerations and Comorbid Insomnia*). Long-term HRT use has declined recently due to its reported association with cardiovascular disease, thrombotic disease, and breast cancer.

■ Insomnia and Pain

The association between pain and sleep problems is evident in **Figure 4.6**. In one survey in Canada, many people with a painful disorder reported sleep problems.[42] The prevalence of insomnia or unrefreshing sleep was related to the severity of pain. In America, the National Sleep Foundation poll in 2003 found that 20% of adults reported pain to disrupt their sleep a few nights a week or more.[38]

Even as painful disease may interfere with sleep, a bidirectional nature is also seen here: several nights of disturbances to the slow-wave (deep) sleep of healthy people induce not only an unrefreshed feeling the next day but also nonspecific generalized muscle aching and fatigue. One such study showed not only this quantitative association, but that pain perception was also a function of sleep quality: poorer sleep resulted in increased somatic attention.[43]

In another study, when patients were deliberately deprived of sleep, their pain sensitivity was also seen to increase. As measured by finger withdrawal from pain, those who slept the least needed less painful pressure to cause reflex removal from the noxious stimulus (**Figure 4.8**). Finally, the situation can become even more complex, as chronic pain and/or the condition that causes it often leads to depression, which itself can contribute to insomnia.

■ Insomnia and Neurologic Diseases

Twenty-five percent of Alzhiemer's patients experience insomnia at some point during their illness.

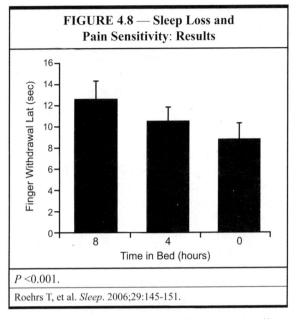

FIGURE 4.8 — Sleep Loss and Pain Sensitivity: Results

$P < 0.001$.

Roehrs T, et al. *Sleep*. 2006;29:145-151.

Moreover, disrupted nocturnal sleep, as well as increased levels of daytime sleepiness, appear to worsen with worsening disease. This has been demonstrated by polysomnograph and actigraphically, as well as by simple behavioral observations.[44] Aberrancies of sleep have been speculated to evolve from gliosis and neuronal loss in the suprachiasmatic nucleus, which have been demonstrated histologically.[45]

Many caregivers of patients with Alzheimer's disease complain of disturbed sleep. Additionally, the physical and emotional stress of caregiving may be related to the development of inflammatory and coagulation responses. In a recent study, caregivers showed higher levels of proinflammatory cytokine interleukin-6 and the procoagulant marker D-dimer. The less total sleep time and poorer sleep efficiency here were thus associated with more inflammation and more coagulability, giving rise to more rates of cardiovascular disease.[39]

Data are emerging on the relationships between sleep and stroke. A recent study showed that the risk of ischemic stroke was increased in men aged 55 to 69 years whose sleep was frequently disturbed. Additionally, significantly higher rates of ischemic heart disease events were found in those with daytime sleepiness.[46] There is also the known association between stroke and sleep-disordered breathing (see Chapter 5, *Common Conditions Associated With Insomnia*). Stroke victims have been shown to experience sleep problems in greater numbers both before and after stroke. In one study, 56.7% of stroke victims reported an insomnia complaint and 37.5% fulfilled the DSM-IV criteria of insomnia. In 38.6%, insomnia had been present prior to the stroke and in 18.1%, it was a consequence of the stroke. What seemed to cause the insomnia after stroke was disability, dementia, anxiety, and use of a psychotropic drug.[47]

A particular type of sleep disturbance has been described in certain patients with Parkinson's disease: dream-enactment behaviors, which represent the absence of normal REM atonia, also referred to as REM sleep behavior disorder. Patients experience aggressive and frightening dreams, and concomitantly flail their arms and vocalize aggressively, at times injuring the bed partner. They are at times known to get out of bed and walk while asleep as they are literally acting out their dreams. However, unlike sleepwalking, these movements are typically purposeful and coordinated, arising out of REM sleep and associated with dream recall. Interestingly, there is suggestion that these sleep symptoms may predate the development of the neurologic manifestations of the disease by more than a decade.[48]

Medications Associated With Insomnia

The list of medications that can interfere with sleep is long (**Table 4.3**).[49-52] The mechanisms by which these medications can alter sleep are varied. The clinician should always consider that the medications the patient is taking may possibly interfere with proper sleep.

Insomnia Due to Poor Sleep Hygiene

Insomnia can be due to impaired sleep hygiene. Characteristics include:

- Duration ≥1 month
- Improper sleep scheduling (frequent daytime napping, variable bedtimes, excessive time in bed)
- Routine use of alcohol, caffeine, or nicotine
- Mentally stimulating, physically activating, or emotionally upsetting activities too close to bedtime
- Frequent use of bed for activities other than sleep
- Uncomfortable sleeping environment.

REFERENCES

1. *Diagnostic and Statistical Manual of Mental Disorders.* 4th ed. Washington, DC: American Psychiatric Association; 2000.

2. International Classification of Sleep Disorders: Diagnostic and Coding Manual. Rochester, Minn: American Sleep Disorders Association; 1990.

3. Ohayon MM, Partinen M. Insomnia and global sleep dissatisfaction in Finland. *J Sleep Res.* 2002;11:339-346.

4. Roth T, Roehrs T. Insomnia: epidemiology, characteristics, and consequences. *Clin Cornerstone.* 2003;5:5-15.

5. Stepanski E, Zorick F, Roehrs T, Young D, Roth T. Daytime alertness in patients with chronic insomnia compared with asymptomatic control subjects. *Sleep.* 1988;11:54-60.

6. Bonnet MH, Arand DL. The consequences of a week of insomnia. *Sleep.* 1996;19:453-461.

7. Bonnet MH, Arand DL. Caffeine use as a model of acute and chronic insomnia. *Sleep.* 1992;15:526-536.

8. Vgontzas AN, Tsigos C, Bixler EO, et al. Chronic insomnia and activity of the stress system: a preliminary study. *J Psychosom Res.* 1998;45:21-31.

9. Richardson GS, Roth T. Future directions in the management of insomnia. *J Clin Psychiatry.* 2001;62(suppl 10):39-45.

10. Spielman AJ, Caruso LS, Glovinsky PB. A behavioral perspective on insomnia treatment. *Psychiatr Clin North Am.* 1987;10:541-553.

11. The New York Times: http://query.nytimes.com/gst/fullpage. html?sec=health&res=9504E7DB1638F934A2575BC0A9659 48260. Accessed December 13, 2006. BBC News: http://news vote.bbc.co.uk/mpapps/pagetools/print/news.bbc.co.uk/1/hi/health/4073897.stm.

12. National Institutes of Health. National Institutes of Health State of the Science Conference Statement on Manifestations and Management of Chronic Insomnia in Adults, June 13-15, 2005. *Sleep.* 2005;28:1049-1057.

13. Doghramji PP. Insomnia in primary care. *Postgraduate Medicine Special Report.* December 2004.

14. Buysse DJ, Reynolds CF 3rd, Kupfer DJ, et al. Clinical diagnoses in 216 insomnia patients using the International Classification of Sleep Disorders (ICSD), DSM-IV and ICD-10 categories: a report from the APA/NIMH DSM-IV Field Trial. *Sleep.* 1994;17:630-637.

15. Ford DE, Kamerow DB. Epidemiologic study of sleep disturbances and psychiatric disorders. An opportunity for prevention? *JAMA.* 1989;262:1479-1484.

TABLE 4.3 — Medications That Can Interfere With Sleep

- Anticholinergics:
  - Agents used to treat Parkinson's disease
  - Ipratropium bromide
- Antihypertensives:
  - β-Blockers (propranolol, atenolol, pindolol)
  - Methyldopa
  - Reserpine
- Antineoplastics:
  - Daunorubicin
  - Goserelin acetate
  - Interferon-α
  - Leuprolide acetate
  - Medroxyprogesterone
  - Pentostatin
- CNS stimulants:
  - Amphetamines
  - Methylphenidate
- Hormones:
  - Cortisone
  - Oral contraceptives
  - Progesterone
  - Thyroid preparations
- Medications that alter CNS neurotransmitters:
  - Amphetamines
  - Antidepressants (tricyclics, monoamine oxidase inhibitors, SSRIs, SNRIs)
  - Antiparkinsonian agents (levodopa, selegiline)
  - Centrally acting antihypertensives (β-blockers, rauwolfia alkaloids, α-agonists)
  - Cholinergic agonists (donepezil, rivastigmine)
  - Quinidine
- Medication withdrawal:
  - Barbiturates
  - Benzodiazepines
  - Ethanol
  - Tricyclics

Continued

- Miscellaneous:
  - Antidepressants
  - Caffeine (Anacin, Excedrin, Empirin, cough/cold preparations)
  - Flutamide (Eulexin)
  - Ketamine (Ketalar)
  - Levodopa
  - Nicotine
  - Phenytoin
  - Quinidine
  - Procarbazine (Matulane)
  - Short-acting barbiturates
- Sympathomimetic amines:
  - Bronchodilators (terbutaline, albuterol, salmeterol, metaproterenol)
  - Decongestants (pseudoephedrine)
  - Xanthine derivatives (theophylline)

Abbreviations: CNS, central nervous system; SNRI, selective norepinephrine reuptake inhibitors; SSRI, selective serotonin reuptake inhibitors.

16. Ohayon MM, Roth T. Place of chronic insomnia in the course of depressive and anxiety disorders. *J Psychiatr Res.* 2003;37:9-15.

17. Breslau N, Roth T, Rosenthal L, Andreski P. Sleep disturbance and psychiatric disorders: a longitudinal epidemiological study of young adults. *Biol Psychiatry.* 1996;39:411-418.

18. Chang PP, Ford DE, Mead LA, Cooper-Patrick L, Klag MJ. Insomnia in young men and subsequent depression. The Johns Hopkins Precursors Study. *Am J Epidemiol.* 1997; 146:105-114.

19. Perlis ML, Giles DE, Buysse DJ, Tu X, Kupfer DJ. Self-reported sleep disturbance as a prodromal symptom in recurrent depression. *J Affect Disord.* 1997;42:209-212.

20. Nierenberg AA, Keefe BR, Leslie VC, et al. Residual symptoms in depressed patients who respond acutely to fluoxetine. *J Clin Psychiatry.* 1999;60:221-225.

21. Agargun MY, Kara H, Solmaz M. Sleep disturbances and suicidal behavior in patients with major depression. *J Clin Psychiatry*. 1997;58:249-251.

22. Fawcett J, Scheftner WA, Fogg L, et al. Time-related predictors of suicide in major affective disorder. *Am J Psychiatry*. 1990;147:1189-1194.

23. Hall RC, Platt DE, Hall RC. Suicide risk assessment: a review of risk factors for suicide in 100 patients who made severe suicide attempts. Evaluation of suicide risk in a time of managed care. *Psychosomatics*. 1999;40:18-27.

24. Fuller KH, Waters WF, Binks PG, Anderson T. Generalized anxiety and sleep architecture: a polysomnographic investigation. *Sleep*. 1997;20:370-376.

25. Saletu-Zyhlarz G, Saletu B, Anderer P, et al. Nonorganic insomnia in generalized anxiety disorder. 1. Controlled studies on sleep, awakening and daytime vigilance utilizing polysomnography and EEG mapping. *Neuropsychobiology*. 1997;36:117-129.

26. Krakow B, Germain A, Tandberg D, et al. Sleep breathing and sleep movement disorders masquerading as insomnia in sexual-assault survivors. *Compr Psychiatry*. 2000;41:49-56.

27. Leibenluft E, Albert PS, Rosenthal NE, Wehr TA. Relationship between sleep and mood in patients with rapid-cycling bipolar disorder. *Psychiatry Res*. 1996;63:161-168.

28. Young DM. Psychiatric morbidity in travelers to Honolulu, Hawaii. *Compr Psychiatry*. 1995;36:224-228.

29. Fawcett JA. Suicide and bipolar disorder. Medscape Psychiatry and Mental Health. 2005;10. Posted August 12, 2005.

30. Monti JM, Monti D. Sleep disturbance in schizophrenia. *Int Rev Psychiatry*. 2005;17:247-253.

31. Corkum P, Tannock R, Moldofsky H. Sleep disturbances in children with attention-deficit/hyperactivity disorder. *J Am Acad Child Adolesc Psychiatry*. 1998;37:637-646.

32. Montano B. Diagnosis and treatment of ADHD in adults in primary care. *J Clin Psychiatry*. 2004;65(suppl 3):18-21.

33. Philipsen A, Feige B, Hesslinger B, et al. Sleep in adults with attention-deficit/hyperactivity disorder: a controlled polysomnographic study including spectral analysis of the sleep EEG. *Sleep*. 2005;28:877-884.

34. Wagner ML, Walters AS, Fisher BC. Symptoms of attention-deficit/hyperactivity disorder in adults with restless legs syndrome. *Sleep*. 2004;27:1499-1504.

35. Cortese S, Konofal E, Lecendreux M, et al. Restless legs syndrome and attention-deficit/hyperactivity disorder: a review of the literature. *Sleep*. 2005;28:1007-1013.

36. Katz DA, McHorney CA. Clinical correlates of insomnia in patients with chronic illness. *Arch Intern Med*. 1998; 158:1099-1107.

37. Dimarino AJ Jr, Banwait KS, Eschinger E, et al. The effect of gastro-oesophageal reflux and omeprazole on key sleep parameters. *Aliment Pharmacol Ther*. 2005;22:325-329.

38. National Sleep Foundation. 2003 Sleep in America Poll. Washington, DC; 2002:1-132.

39. von Kanel R, Dimsdale JE, Ancoli-Israel S, et al. Poor sleep is associated with higher plasma proinflammatory cytokine interleukin-6 and procoagulant marker fibrin D-dimer in older caregivers of people with Alzheimer's disease. *J Am Geriatr Soc*. 2006;54:431-437.

40. National Sleep Foundation. Understanding menopause. Available at: http://www.sleepfoundation.org/hottopics/index.php?secid=17&id+171. Accessed December 13, 2006.

41. Schiff I, Regestein Q, Tulchinsky D, Ryan KJ. Effects of estrogens on sleep and psychological state of hypogonadal women. *JAMA*. 1979;242:2405-2414.

42. Sutton DA, Moldofsky H, Badley EM. Insomnia and health problems in Canadians. *Sleep*. 2001;24:665-670.

43. Affleck G, Urrows S, Tennen H, Higgins P, Abeles M. Sequential daily relations of sleep, pain intensity, and attention to pain among women with fibromyalgia. *Pain*. 1996;68:363-368.

44. Yesavage JA, Friedman L, Ancoli-Israel S, et al. Development of diagnostic criteria for defining sleep disturbance in Alzheimer's disease. *J Geriatr Psychiatry Neurol*. 2003;16:131-139.

45. Stopa EG, Volicer L, Kuo-Leblanc V, et al. Pathologic evaluation of the human suprachiasmatic nucleus in severe dementia. *J Neuropathol Exp Neurol*. 1999;58:29-39.

46. Elwood P, Hack M, Pickering J, Hughes J, Gallacher J. Sleep disturbance, stroke, and heart disease events: evidence from the Caerphilly cohort. *J Epidemiol Community Health*. 2006;60:69-73.

47. Leppavuori A, Pohjasvaara T, Vataja R, Kaste M, Erkinjuntti T. Insomnia in ischemic stroke patients. *Cerebrovasc Dis*. 2002;14:90-97.

48. Schenck CH, Bundlie SR, Mahowald MW. Delayed emergence of a parkinsonian disorder in 38% of 29 older men initially diagnosed with idiopathic rapid eye movement sleep behaviour disorder. *Neurology*. 1996;46:388-393.

49. Kupfer DJ, Reynolds CF 3rd. Management of insomnia. *N Engl J Med*. 1997;336:341-346.

50. Schafer D, Greulich W. Effects of parkinsonian medications on sleep. *J Neurol*. 2000;247(suppl 4):IV24-IV27.

51. Pagel JF, Helfter P. Drug induced nightmares—an etiology based review. *Hum Psychopharmacol*. 2003;18:59-67.

52. Koda-Kimble MA, Young LY, Kradian WA, Guglielmo BJ, Alldredge BK, eds. *Applied Therapeutics: The Clinical Use of Drugs*. 7th edition. Baltimore, Md: Lippincott Williams & Wilkins; 2001:75-20, Section 34.

5

Common Conditions Associated With Insomnia

In this chapter, a heterogeneous group of conditions that often are associated with alterations and disturbances in the structure and quality of sleep will be discussed. These include:

- Sleep-related breathing disorders, such as:
    - Chronic obstructive pulmonary disease (COPD)
    - Sleep apnea syndromes
        - Obstructive sleep apnea syndrome (OSAS)
        - Central sleep apnea syndrome (CSAS)
    - Obesity-hypoventilation syndrome (OHS)
- Restless legs syndrome (RLS)
- Periodic limb movement disorder (PLMD)
- Circadian rhythm sleep disorders, such as:
    - Advanced and delayed sleep-phase syndromes
    - Shift-work sleep disorder (SWSD)
    - Time zone change syndrome (jet lag)
    - Irregular sleep-wake disorder and nonentrained circadian sleep disorder—conditions that are occasionally seen in blind persons and those who are chronically hospitalized.

Sleep-Related Breathing Disorders

Sleep has several effects on breathing, including changes in respiratory control and upper airway resistance. These sleep-related modifications in the respiratory system do not induce adverse effects in healthy subjects, but they may cause problems in patients with various respiratory conditions, including COPD and OHS.[1-3]

■ Chronic Obstructive Pulmonary Disease

Hypoventilation causes the most important gas-exchange alteration during sleep in COPD patients, leading to hypercapnia and hypoxemia, especially during rapid eye movement (REM) sleep when marked respiratory muscle atonia occurs.[4-6] Patients with COPD who are hypoxemic during wakefulness experience an exaggeration of this abnormality during sleep.[7] These alterations in blood gases lead to arousals and awakenings. As a result, symptoms related to sleep disturbances are common in moderate to severe COPD, particularly in elderly patients, in the form of morning tiredness and nocturnal awakenings.

A large survey of patients with COPD found that when one respiratory symptom (cough or wheezing) was present, 39% of patients reported insomnia and 12% reported excessive daytime sleepiness. When both symptoms were present, insomnia and excessive daytime sleepiness were reported by 53% and 23% of patients, respectively.[8]

COPD and OSAS can coexist. Even though the prevalence of OSAS is not greater in COPD patients compared with the general population, the effect of COPD is to produce more profound oxyhemoglobin saturation decrements if it complicates OSAS.[4-7]

Diagnosis and Evaluation

A careful sleep history is the foundation of a diagnosis of sleep-related breathing disorders in COPD patients. Since symptoms related to sleep disturbance are common in patients with moderate to severe COPD and patients notoriously do not volunteer information on sleep problems, patients should be questioned routinely about difficulty falling asleep, staying asleep, middle of the night breathing problems, and medication use at night. Moreover, daytime symptoms should also be clarified, regarding morning tiredness and early awakenings, especially in elderly patients with COPD.[9]

Polysomnography is indicated only in COPD patients who are suspected of having OSAS, or when cor pulmonale and/or polycythemia are not explained by the awake partial pressure of oxygen in arterial blood (PaO_2) level.[10] Patients with mildly diminished PaO_2 levels while awake can develop substantial nocturnal oxygen desaturation, predisposing them to pulmonary hypertension.[11] In such patients, overnight oximetry, rather than full polysomnography, should be considered to determine the extent of nocturnal oxygen desaturation.

Treatment

The first step in treatment of COPD patients with sleep-related breathing disorders is the optimization of underlying therapy for COPD. Pulmonary rehabilitation, particularly inspiratory muscle training, may be useful. For patients with marked daytime hypoxemia (PaO_2 <55-60 mm Hg), continuous O_2 therapy ($\geq$16/24 hours) is the only modality that has been shown to increase survival.[4] In situations of COPD with hypercapnia, higher oxygen flows may cause carbon dioxide retention with resultant morning headache and confusion.[4] This can be remedied by adjusting the O_2 flow rate to maintain the PaO_2 between 60 and 65 mm Hg. Conventional O_2 therapy plus nocturnal noninvasive ventilation can be used in patients with marked hypercapnia.[4] Nocturnal oxygen also should be prescribed to patients who suffer substantial desaturation (sleeping arterial oxygen saturation [SaO_2] <88%) during sleep.[4] This can generally be predicted from daytime hypoxia (PaO_2 <55 mm Hg), and the goal is to maintain arterial oxygen saturation >90% for 70% of the time. Measuring nocturnal oxygen saturation in COPD patients who have daytime PaO_2 of 55-59 mm Hg is not recommended except in patients with unexplained polycythemia or cor pulmonale, in which case oxygen flow should be titrated to maintain PaO_2 $\geq$60 mm Hg.

83

Full polysomnography should be performed in COPD patients whose symptoms suggest coexistent OSAS.

Benzodiazepine receptor agonist (BzRA) hypnotics should be avoided in COPD patients, especially those with hypercapnia and severe COPD. Benzodiazepines decrease upper airway muscle tone and thus increase airway resistance, and they may increase the severity of coexisting OSAS. Also, they may blunt the respiratory drive and enhance SaO_2 decrements during sleep. One study of the use of zolpidem (5 mg to 10 mg) and triazolam (0.25 mg) in patients with mild to moderate COPD revealed that both medications improved sleep quality measures equally. Additionally, as a group, patients did not exhibit a worsening of SaO_2 values or OSAS severity measures while taking either drug when compared with placebo. However, individual patients did reveal a worsening in both variables.[12] Ramelteon is a non-BzRA hypnotic whose mechanism of action is mediated through melatonin receptors. Preliminary evidence suggests that it has no nocturnal respiratory depressant effects in insomnia patients with mild to moderate COPD.[13] However, these results await further confirmation.

The efficacy of treatment with a long-acting inhaled anticholinergic agent was assessed by a recent study by McNicholas and colleagues in a placebo-controlled, double-blind study in patients with severe, stable COPD who were treated for 4 weeks with tiotropium taken in the morning or in the evening.[14] Changes in SaO_2 and sleep quality were assessed. After 4 weeks, FEV_1 correlated with improvement in SaO_2 during REM sleep; however, tiotropium did not change sleep quality.

■ Sleep Apnea Syndrome

The main pathologic entity in sleep apnea syndrome is the repetitive cessation of breathing during sleep. Despite the occurrence of apneas up to hundreds of times during the night, sufferers are typically oblivious to this intermittent suffocation. There are two types of sleep apnea[15]:

- OSAS, in which apnea is mediated through upper airway obstruction
- CSAS, in which apnea is caused by a failure of the respiratory effort during sleep.

In CSAS, the airway is not blocked, but the brain fails to signal the muscles to breathe, possibly owing to instability in the respiratory control center in the brain. CSAS is typically associated with the complaint of disturbed sleep and insomnia, although some patients complain of daytime sleepiness as well. There are many causes of CSAS, but heart failure with systolic dysfunction is the most common. Conversely, many patients with heart failure also have CSAS. The concomitant occurrence of both OSAS and CSAS is more common in congestive heart failure (CHF) than either alone. In a study in which the two were not differentiated, 42 patients with stable CHF and left ventricular dysfunction had an apnea-hypopnea index of ≥ 10 per hour, and 40% to 80% had an apnea-hypopnea index ≥ 15 per hour.[16] CSAS is also observed in the context of central nervous system (CNS) injury from stroke or in neuromuscular diseases, such as amyotrophic lateral sclerosis. Since CSAS is often related to underlying medical conditions, the first step in the management of CSAS is the identification of the underlying cause. Treatment should then be directed at that entity.

OSAS, also known as obstructive sleep apnea/hypopnea syndrome, is the more common of the two forms of apnea. Its main presenting symptoms are excessive daytime sleepiness, snoring, and weight gain. However, insomnia is a presenting symptom in a minority of these patients as well. Patients with OSAS also experience more insomnia. Krell and Kapur assessed the prevalence of insomnia complaints in patients undergoing sleep laboratory evaluation for OSAS. Of 255 consecutive patients with OSAS who underwent polysomnography, 54.9% reported a complaint of insomnia. Of these, 33.4% reported difficulty initiating sleep, 38.8% difficulty maintaining sleep, and 31.4% early morning awakenings.[17]

Despite our limited understanding of its pathophysiology, it is believed to be the result of one or more of the following[15]:

- Anatomic narrowing of the airway
- Increased collapsibility of the airway tissues
- Disturbance in the reflexes that affect the caliber of the upper airway
- Abnormalities of pharyngeal muscle function.

Using the strictest of definitions, OSAS occurs in 2% of women and 4% of men.[18] However, when other risk factors, such as obesity and increasing neck circumference, are present, the prevalence can reach 50%.[19] Even though OSAS was described >30 years ago, most sufferers are undiagnosed, possibly owing to poor public awareness as well as inadequate inquiry regarding its symptoms by medical providers.[20] Meanwhile, the incidence and prevalence of OSAS may be increasing in parallel with the increased prevalence of obesity in the general population as well as in the elderly.[21-23] OSAS contributes to morbidity and mortality, as well as decrements in quality of life. Patients with sleep-disordered breathing have a significantly higher rate of stroke or death from any cause,[24] and the increase is independent of other risk factors, including age, sex, race, body mass index (BMI), hypertension, smoking, and cholesterol levels. Moreover, recent evidence suggests that OSAS is independently associated with *each* of the components of the metabolic syndrome, including obesity, hypertension, glucose intolerance, insulin resistance, and elevated triglycerides; overall, OSAS increases the risk for developing the metabolic syndrome.[25] The many effects of OSAS are illustrated in **Figure 5.1**.

A retrospective chart review analysis by Shepertycky and coworkers found that at the time of OSAS diagnosis, women with OSAS were more likely to be treated for depression, to have insomnia, and to have hypothyroidism than were men with the same degree of OSAS.[26]

Diagnosis

OSAS should be suspected in patients with[27]:

- Family history of OSAS
- History of loud snoring
- Increased BMI (note: 25% of OSAS patients are not obese)
- Large neck size (>17" in men, >16" in women)
- Morning headache
- Morning sore throat or dry mouth
- New-onset unexplained bed-wetting
- Difficulty concentrating and memorizing
- Inappropriate sleepiness (drowsy in passive situations)
- "Crowded" pharynx or any other anatomic reduction in airway size.

Since apneic episodes usually do not result in awakenings and patients are typically unaware of apnea, questioning the patient's bed partner regarding loud snoring, gasping, and trouble breathing is invaluable. Also, there are greater associations between OSAS and the following, and thus suspicion for OSAS should be greater in snorers who have[28]:

- Coronary artery disease, especially prematurely
- Hypertension, especially when resistant
- Stroke
- Polycythemia
- Pulmonary hypertension
- Cor pulmonale

FIGURE 5.1 — Obstructive Sleep Apnea

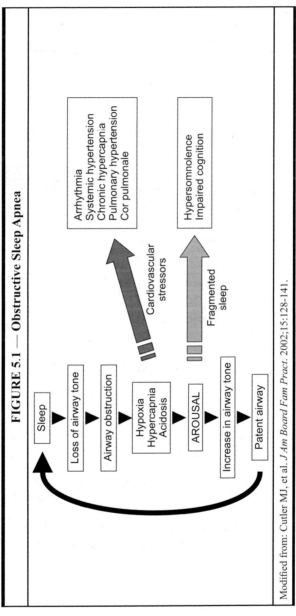

Modified from: Cutler MJ, et al. *J Am Board Fam Pract.* 2002;15:128-141.

- Morning and nocturnal headaches
- CHF
- Arrhythmias
- Nocturnal angina.

When OSAS is suspected, patients should be referred to a sleep laboratory for polysomnography. This is the only currently accepted confirmatory test. It is used not only to confirm the diagnosis and determine OSAS severity (measured as the apnea-hypopnea index [AHI] expressed as the frequency of apneic episodes/hour of sleep) but also to assess treatment efficacy.

Treatment

Depending on the severity of OSAS and its clinical and functional impact, treatment ranges from conservative measures to surgical interventions[29]:

- Measures that can be implemented rapidly (within a few days or weeks):
  - Avoidance of CNS depressants
  - Positioning: sleeping on one side (sewing a few tennis balls to the back of a T-shirt) can reduce AHI up to 50% in patients who exhibit an exacerbation of the AHI while lying in the supine position[30-32]
  - Continuous positive airway pressure (cPAP) or bilevel positive airway pressure (BiPAP)
- Measures whose implementation requires prolonged periods of time (months):
  - Dental appliances (**Figure 5.2**)
  - Weight loss: especially when OSAS developed after significant weight gain
  - Surgery: uvulopalatopharyngopalatoplasty, laser-assisted uvuloplasty, tonsillectomy and adenoidectomy, nasal polypectomy, septoplasty, mandibular advancement osteotomy, and tracheostomy, among others (**Figure 5.3**).

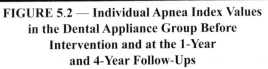

FIGURE 5.2 — Individual Apnea Index Values in the Dental Appliance Group Before Intervention and at the 1-Year and 4-Year Follow-Ups

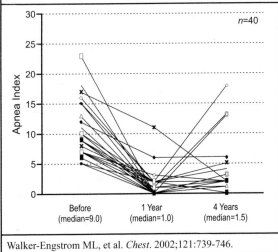

Walker-Engstrom ML, et al. *Chest*. 2002;121:739-746.

Overweight patients can benefit from weight reduction. Weight loss of as little as 10% reduced the frequency of apneic events by 26% in one study.[33] Individuals with OSAS should avoid CNS suppressants (eg, alcohol and sedative/hypnotics), which make the airway more likely to collapse during sleep and prolong the apneic periods. Smoking cessation is important since cigarette smoke can increase the swelling in the upper airway, which may worsen both snoring and apnea. Since apneic episodes occur in some patients with mild sleep apnea syndrome only when they sleep on their backs, using pillows and other devices that help them sleep in a side position may be helpful.

For patients with moderate to severe OSAS, cPAP is considered first-line treatment. It consists of an ambulatory device that introduces air at a high pressure into

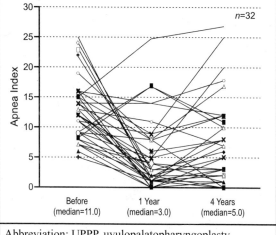

FIGURE 5.3 — Individual Apnea Index Values in the UPPP Group Before Intervention and at the 1-Year and 4-Year Follow-Ups

n=32

Apnea Index

Before (median=11.0)   1 Year (median=3.0)   4 Years (median=5.0)

Abbreviation: UPPP, uvulopalatopharyngoplasty.

Walker-Engstrom ML, et al. *Chest*. 2002;121:739-746.

the nares, mouth, or both during sleep. The air pressure should be adjusted in a sleep laboratory so that it is just enough to prevent the upper airway tissues from collapsing during sleep. While cPAP prevents airway closure while in use, apnea episodes return when cPAP is discontinued or used improperly. Other types of devices that vary in the way in which pressure is delivered are also available for people having difficulty tolerating cPAP, such as BiPAP, in which the inspiratory pressure is lower than the expiratory pressure.

Patients who are receiving chronic treatment with BiPAP or cPAP should be referred to the sleep disorders center if they have a return of sleepiness or snoring while using these devices, if they gain substantial amounts of weight, if they have major changes in medical status (ie, myocardial infarction or stroke), or if noncompliance is suspected. Patients should be urged to keep in close contact with home care companies to ensure that they receive assistance in case of worn-out mask and tubing, malfunctioning machines, etc.

The mandibular advancement device is the most widely used dental appliance for OSAS. Others include the anterior mandibular positioning dental device. Both devices force the lower jaw forward and down slightly, thus keeping the airway open, similar in principle to the "jaw-thrust" maneuver in cardiac and pulmonary rehabilitation. Both have been found to be successful in some individuals, yet their overall efficacy rate is lower than that of cPAP. Their main side effects are dry lips, tooth discomfort, excessive salivation, and pain that awakens users, enough so that half of patients discontinue device use. Moreover, long-term use has caused permanent changes in the position of the teeth or jaw; therefore, regular visits to dental professionals are warranted.

There are several surgical procedure options, outpatient and inpatient. Surgery may be of benefit for patients with upper airway obstruction, such as a deviated nasal septum, markedly enlarged tonsils, or small lower jaw with an overbite, causing the throat to be abnormally narrow. These procedures are typically performed after OSAS has failed to respond to conservative measures and a trial of cPAP.

A substantial number of patients appropriately treated for OSAS have residual excessive sleepiness.[34] Possible causes include:

- Inadequate total sleep time due to voluntary reasons
- Inadequate cPAP pressure
- Coexistent illnesses or medications
- Coexistent RLS/PLMD or narcolepsy
- Depression, anxiety, other psychiatric illness
- Hypoxic brain injury prior to cPAP.

Remedies for these include:

- Increasing total sleep time
- Addressing underlying medical and psychiatric conditions
- Sleep hygiene
- Pharmacologic aids in initiating and maintaining sleep (only when cPAP is in use)
- Optimize cPAP therapy (commonly left up to the sleep laboratory and its ancillary respiratory department)
  - Check mask fit/type
  - Adjust pressure
- Treat rhinitis/sinusitis and nasal obstruction.

If residual sleepiness persists despite adequate compliance with cPAP, and if no other underlying cause can be detected, modafinil has been shown to reduce the excessive daytime sleepiness in patients with OSAS. Its putative mechanism is increased activity in the tuberomammillary nucleus in the hypothalamus. It does not diminish the apnea severity; it is a treatment for residual sleepiness only. Specifics regarding the use of modafinil include:

- Usual dose: 200-400 mg/day
- Potential drug-drug interactions via CYP 2C9; mild induction of 1A2, 3A4, 2B6
- Side effects (dose-related) include headache, nausea, nervousness, anorexia, and dry mouth.

■ Obesity-Hypoventilation Syndrome

Although a patient with this disorder typically does not present with the symptom of insomnia, it is being discussed in this chapter since it represents a disordered breathing during sleep and can complicate the sleep of insomnia patients. OHS was initially identified 50 years ago as the Pickwickian syndrome. The clinical presentation of patients with OHS may include symptoms such as excessive daytime sleepiness, fatigue, or morning headache, similar to symptoms seen with OSAS. Although the prevalence of OSAS among obese people is ~40% (conversely, ~70% of people with OSAS are obese), unlike OSAS patients, patients with OHS have daytime hypoxemia and hypercapnea.[35] Thus patients with OHS may present with a spectrum of sleep-related breathing disorders and sleep disturbances due to restriction of ventilatory function, sleep-induced hypoxemia, and/or hypercapnea, or both.[35,36]

Diagnosis

The identification and treatment of patients with OHS is important since untreated patients may develop secondary erythrocytosis and will ultimately develop pulmonary hypertension and cor pulmonale.[35] The diagnostic criteria for OHS are shown in **Table 5.1**.

Evaluations should include:

- Arterial blood gas testing to confirm daytime hypercapnea
- Complete blood count (CBC) to determine existence of erythrocytosis
- Serum electrolytes
- Identification of conditions that aggravate chronic hypoventilation (eg, excessive use of alcohol, sedative-hypnotics, or narcotics)
- Pulmonary function testing to determine presence/severity of COPD
- Nighttime polysomnography if there is a suspicion of sleep disorders, such as OSAS.

TABLE 5.1 — Diagnostic Criteria for Obesity-Hypoventilation Syndrome

- Body mass index ≥ 30 kg/m^2
- Daytime PaCO$_2$ >45 mm Hg
- Associated sleep-related breathing disorder (obstructive sleep apnea or sleep hypoventilation or both)
- Absence of other known causes of hypoventilation

Treatment

The ideal treatment of OHS is weight loss, which can improve most of the underlying physiologic abnormalities. However, weight loss is slow to occur and difficult to maintain. Therefore, in some cases, gastric surgery may be indicated.[35,37]

As noted previously, patients with OHS can have a variety of sleep-related disturbances. Therefore, treatment that corrects the individual's sleep-related breathing problems should be used. For example:

- In patients with concurrent OSAS, cPAP (via nasal mask) is usually effective, although a subset of patients may not respond, necessitating noninvasive mechanical ventilation to alleviate hypercapnea.
- In patients whose underlying sleep disorder is hypoventilation alone, noninvasive mechanical ventilation is the mainstay of treatment.

Restless Legs Syndrome (RLS)

Restless legs syndrome is a neurologic disorder of uncertain etiology characterized by unpleasant sensations deep inside the legs. These paresthesias are often difficult for the patient to describe, but terms used include "creepy, crawly, pulling, crampy, tingling, weird pain, electric, stinging, tension, itching, nervousness, growing pains, and burning." They can be felt anywhere in the legs but most commonly in the calves. These symptoms worsen as the day progresses and are most pronounced when the patient is going to bed. The hallmark feature is the basis for its name: an irresistible urge to move the legs, which results in a temporary relief of the paresthesia.

When RLS is advanced, a person may feel these symptoms in the hands and arms as well. Because RLS typically occurs in the evening and while one is sleeping, it causes difficulty falling asleep and even staying asleep. Symptoms typically peak between midnight and 4 AM; however, the circadian rhythm nature of the symptoms persists even in "unconventional" sleep/wake cycles (eg, in shift workers). When symptoms are very severe, the worsening at night may not be noticeable but must have been previously present in order for it to be considered RLS. Diagnostic and ancillary symptoms of the disorder are listed in **Table 5.2** and **Table 5.3**. Despite the discomfort in all cases, most patients consider sleep-related RLS symptoms to be most troublesome (**Figure 5.4**).[38]

Epidemiologic studies indicate that RLS is present in about 5% to 10% of the general population.[39] However, many patients with RLS often go undiagnosed or misdiagnosed.[40] The mean age at onset of RLS is 27.2 years, but prevalence increases with age. Interestingly, the onset is before age 20 in 38.3% of patients.[41]

RLS can be either idiopathic or secondary to other conditions[42]:

- Idiopathic:
  - Most common form (75% of patients)
  - Familial: 92% report family history
  - Autosomal dominant inheritance is suspected
  - Incidence increases with age
- Secondary:
  - Uremia (20% to 40% of dialysis patients)
  - Iron storage deficiency
  - Polyneuropathy (especially diabetic peripheral neuropathy)
  - Pregnancy (up to 27%)
  - Fibromyalgia
  - Rheumatoid arthritis
  - Sjögren's syndrome
  - Radiculopathy
  - Folate deficiency
  - Attention-deficit/hyperactivity disorder (ADHD)

TABLE 5.2 — IRLSSG Essential Diagnostic Criteria

- Urge to move legs (arms, other body parts) with or without uncomfortable/unpleasant sensations in the legs
- Begins or worsens during periods of rest or inactivity (lying, sitting)
- Partially or totally relieved by movement (walking, stretching)
- Worse in the evening or night

Abbreviation: IRLSSG, International Restless Legs Syndrome Study Group.

Adapted from: Allen RP, et al. *Sleep Med.* 2003;4:101-119.

TABLE 5.3 — IRLSSG Nonessential But Common Features

- Family history; prevalence in first-degree relatives 3 to 5 times greater than in those without RLS
- Response to dopaminergic therapy
- Periodic limb movements during sleep or wakefulness
- Variable clinical course
- Sleep disturbance
- Medical/physical evaluation in primary RLS reveals no abnormalities

Abbreviations: IRLSSG, International Restless Legs Syndrome Study Group; RLS, restless legs syndrome.

Adapted from: Allen RP, et al. *Sleep Med.* 2003;4:101-119.

 — Medications: dopamine antagonists, tricyclic antidepressants, selective serotonin reuptake inhibitors, lithium, and xanthines.

A telephone-interview poll conducted by the National Sleep Foundation in 2005 in a random, representative sample of US adults found that 9.7% reported symptoms of RLS that included unpleasant feelings in the legs for at least a few nights a week, which were

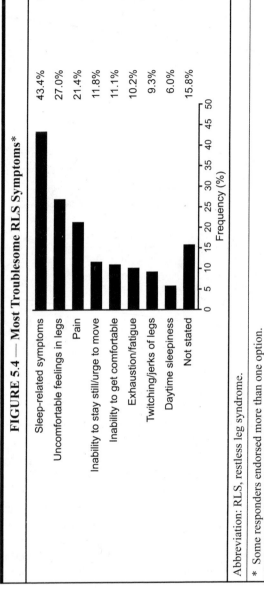

FIGURE 5.4 — Most Troublesome RLS Symptoms*

Symptom	Frequency (%)
Sleep-related symptoms	43.4%
Uncomfortable feelings in legs	27.0%
Pain	21.4%
Inability to stay still/urge to move	11.8%
Inability to get comfortable	11.1%
Exhaustion/fatigue	10.2%
Twitching/jerks of legs	9.3%
Daytime sleepiness	6.0%
Not stated	15.8%

Abbreviation: RLS, restless leg syndrome.

* Some responders endorsed more than one option.

Hening W, et al. *Sleep Med.* 2004;5:237-246.

worse at bedtime.[43] In another study in a large primary care population, weekly RLS symptoms were reported by 9.6% of study subjects, most of whom reported impaired sleep consistent with a diagnosis of insomnia.[40] Follow-up questionnaires completed by their primary care physicians indicated that only 37.9% of these individuals had consulted with them about their RLS symptoms, and a diagnosis of RLS was given in only 25% of cases.

■ Pathophysiology of Primary RLS

Even though the cause is unknown, RLS is believed be related to dopaminergic dysfunction[44] as well as decreased iron storage in the CSF.[45] Pharmacologic evidence that RLS is highly responsive to dopaminergic agents suggests the former. Furthermore, the symptoms of RLS and PLMD are worse during the night, a time when the circadian levels of dopamine are at their lowest.[46] Reduced ferritin and elevated transferrin levels in the cerebrospinal fluid (CSF) indicate that patients with RLS possess low brain iron levels.[45,47,48]

■ Diagnosis

The diagnosis of RLS is based on a thorough history and physical examination. Patients presenting with insomnia and/or tiredness should be questioned regarding uncomfortable symptoms in their limbs that worsen at night and that are relieved by movement. A neurologic exam is important to rule out Parkinson's disease, neuropathy, and weakness. Polysomnography is not generally indicated in evaluation of RLS. Appropriate laboratory tests include serum CBC, iron, total iron-binding capacity (TIBC), and ferritin level. Low ferritin levels, even with no anemia and normal circulating iron levels, are related to RLS. Moreover, even though most normal laboratory values for ferritin start at 10 mcg/L, patients with ferritin levels <50 mcg/L should be considered for iron treatment.[49]

Other screening tests include folate, cobalamin, blood urea nitrogen (BUN)/creatinine, and fasting blood glucose (FBG), as well as other tests for potential secondary causes, if suspected. A complete medication history is also important to determine if the patient is using those associated with RLS (eg, dopamine agonists).

Although about 80% of people who have RLS have periodic limb movements (PLMs),[41] the presence of PLMs is neither necessary nor sufficient to make the diagnosis of RLS.

The severity of RLS symptoms can be assessed with the 10-question International Restless Legs Syndrome Study Group (**Table 5.4**).[50] The patient must rate his or her symptoms on a scale of 0 to 4, with 0

TABLE 5.4 — IRLSSG Rating Scale

1. Overall, how would you rate the RLS discomfort in your legs or arms?
2. Overall, how would you rate the need to move around because of your RLS symptoms?
3. Overall, how much relief of your RLS arm or leg discomfort do you get from moving around?
4. Overall, how severe is your sleep disturbance from your RLS symptoms?
5. How severe is your tiredness or sleepiness from your RLS symptoms?
6. Overall, how severe is your RLS as a whole?
7. How often (days/week) do you get RLS symptoms?
8. When you have RLS symptoms, how severe (number of hours) are they in an average day?
9. Overall, how severe is the impact of your RLS symptoms on your ability to carry out your daily affairs?
10. How severe is your mood disturbance from your RLS symptoms?

Abbreviations: IRLSSG, International Restless Legs Syndome Study Group; RLS, restless legs syndrome.

Adapted from: Walters AS, et al. *Sleep Med.* 2003;4:121-132.

representing "none" and 4 representing "very severe." This is a useful questionnaire to use when following patients who are undergoing treatment.

■ **Treatment**

The treatment of RLS obviously should first address the possibility of secondary causes, including discontinuation of medications that can cause or exacerbate the condition. If the diagnosis is idiopathic RLS, treatment can vary, depending on the frequency and intensity of the symptoms. However, even before medication choice is made, establishing and maintaining good sleep hygiene may diminish symptoms, although this has yet to be subjected to empiric validation. Other measures include using an ice pack or heating pad, taking a warm bath, and exercising briefly (eg, running in place) before bedtime. These measures may provide temporary relief. Caffeine and alcohol should be avoided. Pharmacologic therapy is used for symptomatic relief and is not curative. First-line medications traditionally have included dopamine agonist agents, such as pramipexole, pergolide, levodopa, and ropinirole. Ropinirole is the only one of these currently approved by the Food and Drug Administration (FDA) for treatment of the symptoms of RLS.[51]

Analgesics, antiepileptics, benzodiazepines, and benzodiazepine-like hypnotics have also been used, but results of trials have at times been conflicting. These compounds are also not indicated by the FDA for the disorder.

Periodic Limb Movement Disorder

PLMD is a neurologic motor condition characterized by stereotype, periodic jerking movements typically consisting of flexion of the ankle, knee, and hip. Unlike RLS, PLMD is rarely diagnosed in patients under the age of 30 but is found in 44% of patients aged 65 and older. Frequently unnoticed by patients, these involuntary movements occur periodically throughout the night and are sometimes accompanied by awakenings, leading to the complaint of insomnia or daytime sleepiness. They tend to cluster in episodes that last anywhere from a few minutes to several hours and can fluctuate in severity from one night to the next. These movements are very different from nocturnal leg cramps, which are painful spasms of the calf or foot that are often experienced initially while falling asleep. These occur with greater frequency during pregnancy, in women, in the elderly, after intense exercise, as a result of diabetes, with fluid and electrolyte imbalances, and with musculoskeletal disorders. There is some relationship between PLMD and RLS, and some investigators consider the two to be the same condition. PLMs are so common in RLS that they are considered to be supportive of an RLS diagnosis when other RLS symptoms are present; conversely, up to 80% of those with RLS also experience PLMs.[52]

The causes of PLMD are unknown. However, recent research has shown that people with a variety of medical problems, including Parkinson's disease and narcolepsy, may have frequent PLMs in sleep. PLMD may be induced by medications, most notably, antidepressants. In fact, given that many normal physiologic changes that occur with aging, such as reduced muscle mass and diminished skin elasticity, perhaps the higher prevalence of PLMD in the elderly actually represents a normal function of aging as opposed to a true sleep disorder.

■ **Diagnosis**

While RLS is a diagnosis made essentially via symptomatology, PLMD is diagnosed via testing. PLMD should be suspected in patients who complain of insomnia as well as daytime sleepiness. A sleep partner may observe the occurrence of PLMs, which often affect the partner before the patient knows of his or her behavior. However, definitive diagnosis of PLMD requires overnight polysomnography. Laboratory studies to assess iron status, folic acid, vitamin B_{12}, thyroid function, and magnesium levels can be helpful in identifying secondary causes.

■ Treatment

Since caffeine often intensifies the symptoms of PLMD, caffeine-containing products, such as chocolate, coffee, tea, and soft drinks, should be avoided. Generally, treatment of PLMD overlaps that for RLS. Although no medication is specifically FDA-indicated for PLMs, certain medications have been utilized, including the dopamine agonists, anticonvulsant medications, and benzodiazepines.[53] As with RLS, current first-line treatment recommendations are the anti-Parkinson's medications.

Circadian Rhythm Sleep Disorders

A variety of sleep disorders are characterized by a persistent or recurrent pattern of sleep disruption that is due to a mismatching between the sleep/wake schedule required or desired by a person's environment or lifestyle and their circadian sleep/wake pattern. To be diagnosed with this disorder, this mismatch must:

- Lead to excessive insomnia or daytime sleepiness
- Cause clinically important distress or impair work or social life.

Also, the insomnia cannot occur solely during a psychiatric disorder or another sleep disorder and it is not directly caused by a general medical condition or substance use, including prescription medications and drugs of abuse.

■ Delayed Sleep-Phase Syndrome

In this circadian rhythm disorder, the onset of the major sleep episode is *delayed* by ≥2 hours of the desired clock time. An example of this syndrome would be in the case of someone whose desired regular schedule is to go to bed at 10 or 11 PM and get up at 7 or 8 AM but who consistently has difficulty in falling asleep, regardless of use of sleep aids, until 1 or 2 AM, then finds it hard to get up at the desired time. In such cases, the individual's circadian rhythm is out of phase with their daily routine.

Adolescence appears to be the most common period of life for the onset of this sleep disorder.

Treatment

Treatment of this syndrome would typically be indicated if it persists for ≥3 months and leads to impairment in social or occupational functioning. Specific treatment options include:
- Bright-light therapy
- Chronotherapy
- Melatonin.

Bright-light therapy requires exposure of the patient to a light box that emits 2,500 to 10,000 lux of full-spectrum light for 2 hours upon the patient's arising in the early morning. Patients must also avoid light in the evening. A phase advance of the person's circadian rhythm typically occurs after about 1 week.

Chronotherapy is a behavioral technique in which bedtime and final awakening time are systematically delayed by 3-hour increments. This procedure is maintained until the desired bedtime is reached (eg, 11 PM). Once a normal rhythm is established, patients must strictly adhere to these sleep times to avoid a recurrence of the syndrome.

Melatonin, a pineal gland hormone whose secretion is inhibited by light and enhanced during darkness, plays a major role in regulating circadian rhythms in animals. Administration to humans at available doses (0.5-10 mg daily 1 hour before bedtime) produces supraphysiologic levels. Melatonin can affect phase-shifting circadian rhythms in patients with many of the circadian rhythm disorders; the strongest indication for its use is in delayed sleep-phase syndrome.[54] Since the insomnia associated with circadian rhythm disorders is the sleep-initiation variety, the melatonin receptor agonist ramelteon (see Chapter 9, *Pharmacologic Agents for Insomnia*) may also be useful for initiating phase shifting similar to that with melatonin. However, clinical data on the use of ramelteon for this type of insomnia is currently lacking.

■ Advanced Sleep-Phase Syndrome

In this circadian rhythm disorder, the major sleep episode is *advanced* by ≥2 hours of the desired clock time, which results in the inability to stay awake until the desired bedtime or the inability to remain asleep until the desired arising time. Unlike other sleep-maintenance disorders, the early morning awakening occurs after a normal amount of undisturbed sleep. Typical sleep-onset times are between 6 and 9 PM, and awakening times are between 3 and 5 AM.

The advanced sleep-phase syndrome is more likely to appear in the elderly.

Treatment

The treatment options for the advanced sleep-phase syndrome are the same as in the delayed sleep-phase syndrome, namely:

- Bright-light therapy
- Chronotherapy
- Melatonin.

■ Time Zone Change Syndrome

More commonly called "jet lag," this circadian rhythm disorder is characterized by varying degrees of difficulty in initiating or maintaining sleep, excessive sleepiness, decrements in subjective daytime performance, and somatic complaints (eg, headaches, altered appetite, and gastrointestinal function) following rapid travel across multiple time zones.

Prevention

Several strategies can help avoid or minimize the symptoms of jet lag. In general, it is important to begin to adapt to the routine of the travel destination as soon as boarding the flight, which should include:

- Resetting watches and clocks for the new time zone upon boarding the plane
- Avoiding long or inappropriate naps (eg, limiting sleep to no more than 2 hours immediately after arrival, avoiding going to sleep immediately after an overnight flight)
- Exposure to daylight (taking a 1-hour walk) as soon as possible after awakening
- Avoiding excessive caffeine and alcohol.

■ Shift-Work Sleep Disorder

This sleep disorder affects people who frequently rotate shifts or work at night. Schedules of these people go against the body's natural circadian rhythm, and individuals have difficulty adjusting to this different schedule. SWSD consists of a constant or recurrent pattern of sleep interruption that results in insomnia or excessive sleepiness. Other symptoms and consequences of SWSD include:

- Difficulty concentrating
- Headaches
- Lack of energy
- Increased accidents

- Increased work-related errors
- Increased sick leave.

Treatment

Unfortunately, treatment for SWSD is limited. Both behavioral and pharmacologic remedies can help alleviate symptoms. Some research indicates that the body may never fully adapt to shift work, especially for those who switch to a normal weekend sleep schedule. Some strategies for adequate restorative sleep include:

- Wearing dark glasses to block out the sunlight on the way home
- Keeping to the same bedtime and waking time schedule, even on weekends
- Eliminating noise and light from the sleep environment (use eye masks and ear plugs)
- Avoiding caffeinated beverages and foods close to bedtime
- Avoiding alcohol; although it may seem to improve sleep initially, tolerance develops quickly and it soon disturbs sleep.

The wake-promoting agent modafinil is the one medication approved for excessive sleepiness associated with SWSD. In SWSD, the drug improves nighttime wakefulness without disrupting daytime sleep. Modafinil is generally well tolerated by patients and has a low abuse potential. It is usually prescribed in doses of 200 mg to 400 mg taken 1 hour before beginning the work shift; once established, the timing of the dose should not be changed.[55]

■ Sleep Disorders and Blindness

Blind individuals are not only handicapped by their loss of vision, but are also affected because the loss of sight, and therefore exposure to day/night light changes, can have a secondary impact on their circadian rhythm.

Most totally blind people have circadian rhythm that is "free running" (ie, that is not synchronized to environmental time cues and that oscillates on a cycle slightly longer than 24 hours). This condition causes recurrent insomnia and daytime sleepiness when the rhythm drifts out of phase with the normal 24-hour cycle.[56]

A prospective questionnaire survey of 1500 blind individuals and 1000 sighted controls found that individuals evaluated as being totally blind or almost blind (ie, <10% vision in only one eye) reported a significantly higher occurrence of sleep/wake disorders than did controls.[57] Nocturnal sleep disruption and daytime somnolence were significantly more common in blind individuals. In addition, there was an increased use of sleeping pills and a higher incidence of involuntary daily naps.

In a more recent study, Leger and colleagues polygraphically monitored 26 blind individuals with no light perception and free-running melatonin rhythms and compared the results with those from matched controls.[58] Total sleep time, sleep latency, sleep efficiency, and total REM sleep were significantly lower in the blind subjects than in matched controls.

Treatment

The influence of light on circadian rhythm, and hence on the timing of sleep, is assumed to be mediated by melatonin, a hormone of the pineal gland, whose secretion is inhibited by light and enhanced during darkness. Fischer and associates performed a double-blind crossover study in totally blind individuals to determine whether a single administration of melatonin would improve sleep and associated neuroendocrine patterns.[59] Subjects received 5 mg melatonin or placebo orally 1 hour before bedtime. Administration of exogenous melatonin increased blood melatonin concentrations to supraphysiologic levels, significantly increased total sleep time and sleep efficiency, and reduced time awake. The increase in total sleep time was primarily due to an increase in stage 2 sleep and a slight increase in REM sleep. In addition, melatonin normalized in parallel the temporal pattern of ACTH and cortisol plasma concentration. Several other studies have shown that continuing administration of melatonin at doses of 0.5 to 10 mg/day can entrain the circadian rhythms in most blind people who have a free-running circadian rhythm and result in improvements in a number of sleep parameters.[54,56,60]

In addition to the use of melatonin, some research suggests that the regular timing of other activities, including exercise and eating, may help entrain the circadian rhythm.[61]

REFERENCES

1. Iber C. Sleep-related breathing disorders. *Neurol Clin.* 2005;23:1045-1057.

2. Lewis KL. Apneas, hypopneas, and respiratory effort-related arousals: moving closer to a standard. *Curr Opin Pulm Med.* 2002;8:493-497.

3. Fanfulla F, Cascone L, Taurino AE. Sleep disordered breathing in patients with chronic obstructive pulmonary disease. *Minerva Med.* 2004;95:307-321.

4. Mohsenin V. Sleep in chronic obstructive pulmonary disease. *Semin Respir Crit Care Med.* 2005;26:109-116.

5. Kutty K. Sleep and chronic obstructive pulmonary disease. *Curr Opin Pulm Med.* 2004;10:104-112.

6. Gay PC. Chronic obstructive pulmonary disease and sleep. *Respir Care.* 2004;49:39-51.

7. Weitzenblum E, Chaouat A. Sleep and chronic obstructive pulmonary disease. *Sleep Med Rev.* 2004;8:281-294.

8. Klink ME, Dodge R, Quan SF. The relation of sleep complaints to respiratory symptoms in a general population. *Chest.* 1994;105:151-154.

9. Bellia V, Catalano F, Scichilone N, et al. Sleep disorders in the elderly with and without chronic airflow obstruction: the SARA study. *Sleep.* 2003;26:318-323.

10. McNicholas WT. Impact of sleep in COPD. *Chest.* 2000;117(suppl 2):48S-53S.

11. Fletcher EC, Luckett RA, Miller T, Costarangos C, Lurka N, Fletcher JG. Pulmonary vascular hemodynamics in chronic lung disease patients with and without oxyhemoglobin desaturation during sleep. *Chest.* 1989;95:757-764.

12. Steens RD, Pouliot Z, Millar TW, Kryger MH, George CF. Effects of zolpidem and triazolam on sleep and respiration in mild to moderate chronic obstructive pulmonary disease. *Sleep.* 1993;16:318-326.

13. Sainati S, Tsymbalov S, Demissie S, Roth T. Double-blind, placebo-controlled, two-way crossover study of ramelteon in subjects with mild to moderate chronic obstructive pulmonary disease (COPD). *Sleep.* 2005;28(suppl):A162.

14. McNicholas WT, Calverley PM, Lee A, et al. Long-acting inhaled anticholinergic therapy improves sleeping oxygen saturation in COPD. *Eur Respir J.* 2004;23:825-831.

15. Gottlieb DJ. Can sleep apnea be treated without modifying anatomy? *N Engl J Med.* 2005;353:2604-2606.

16. Javaheri S, Parker TJ, Wexler L, et al. Occult sleep-disordered breathing in stable congestive heart failure. *Ann Intern Med.* 1995;122:487-492.

17. Krell SB, Kapur VK. Insomnia complaints in patients evaluated for obstructive sleep apnea. *Sleep Breath.* 2005;9:104-110.

18. Young T, Palta M, Dempsey J, Skatrud J, Weber S, Badr S. The occurrence of sleep-disordered breathing among middle-aged adults. *N Engl J Med.* 1993;328:1230-1235.

19. Resta OL, Foschino-Barbaro MP, Legari G, et al., Sleep-related breathing disorders, loud snoring and excessive daytime sleepiness in obese subjects. *Int J Obes Relat Metab Disord.* 2001;25:669-675.

20. Redline S, Strohl KP. Recognition and consequences of obstructive sleep apnea hypopnea syndrome. *Clin Chest Med.* 1998;19:1-19.

21. Flegal KM, Carroll MD, Ogden CL, Johnson CL. Prevalence and trends in obesity among US adults, 1999-2000. *JAMA.* 2002;288:1723-1727.

22. Mokdad AH, Serdula MK, Dietz WH, Bowman BA, Marks JS, Koplan JP. The spread of the obesity epidemic in the United States, 1991-1998. *JAMA.* 1999;282:1519-1522.

23. Arterburn DE, Crane PK, Sullivan SD. The coming epidemic of obesity in elderly Americans. *J Am Geriatr Soc.* 2004; 52:1907-1912.

24. Shahar E, Whitney CW, Redline S, et al. Sleep-disordered breathing and cardiovascular disease: cross-sectional results of the Sleep Heart Health Study. *Am J Respir Crit Care Med.* 2001;163:19-25.

25. Coughlin SR, Mawdsley L, Mugarza JA, Calverley PM, Wilding JP. Obstructive sleep apnoea is independently associated with an incrased prevalence of metabolic syndrome. *Eur Heart J.* 2004;25:735-741.

26. Shepertycky MR, Banno K, Kryger MH. Differences between men and women in the clinical presentation of patients diagnosed with obstructive sleep apnea syndrome. *Sleep.* 2005;28:309-314.

27. Skomro RP, Kryger MH. Clinical presentations of obstructive sleep apnea syndrome. *Prof Cardiovasc Dis.* 1999;41:331-340.

28. Flemons WW. Clinical practice. Obstructive sleep apnea. *N Engl J Med.* 2002;347:498-504.

29. Morin CM. Psychological and behavioral treatments for primary insomnia. In: Kryger MH, Roth T, Dement WC, eds. *Principles and Practice of Sleep Medicine.* 4th ed. Philadephia, Pa: WB Saunders; 2005:726-737.

5

30. Pevernagie DA, Stanson AW, Sheedy PF 2nd, Daniels BK, Shepard JW Jr. Effects of body position on the upper airway of patients with obstructive sleep apnea. *Am J Respir Crit Care Med.* 1995;152:179-185.

31. Cartwright R, Ristanovic R, Diaz F, Caldarelli D, Alder G. A comparative study of treatments for positional sleep apnea. *Sleep.* 1991;14:546-552.

32. Pevernagie DA, Shepard JW Jr. Relations between sleep stage, posture and effective nasal CPAP levels in OSA. *Sleep.* 1992;15:162-167.

33. Peppard PE, Young T, Palta M, Dempsey J, Skatrud J. Longitudinal study of moderate weight change and sleep-disordered breathing. *JAMA.* 2000;284:3015-3021.

34. Patel SR, White DP, Malhotra A, Stanchina ML, Ayas NT. Continuous positive airway pressure therapy for treating sleepiness in a diverse population with obstructive sleep apnea: results of a meta-analysis. *Arch Intern Med.* 2003;163:565-571.

35. Olson AL, Zwillich C. The obesity hypoventilation syndrome. *Am J Med.* 2005;118:948-1056.

36. Poulin M, Doucet M, Major GC, et al. The effect of obesity on chronic respiratory diseases: pathophysiology and therapeutic strategies. *CMAJ.* 2006;174:1230-1239.

37. Berger KI, Ayappa I, Chatr-Amontri B, et al. Obesity hypoventilation syndrome as a spectrum of respiratory disturbances during sleep. *Chest.* 2001;120:1231-1238.

38. Hening WA. Restless legs syndrome: the most common and least diagnosed sleep disorder. *Sleep Med.* 2004;5:429-430.

39. Phillips B, Young T, Finn L, Asher K, Kening WA, Purvis C. Epidemiology of restless legs symptoms in adults. *Arch Intern. Med.* 2000;160:2137-2141.

40. Hening W, Walters AS, Allen RP, et al. Impact, diagnosis and treatment of restless legs syndrome (RLS) in a primary care population: the REST (RLS epidemiology, symptoms, and treatment) primary care study. *Sleep Medicine.* 2004;5:237-246.

41. Montplaisir J, Boucher S, Poirier G, Lavigne G, Lapierre O, Lesperance P. Clinical, polysomnographic, and genetic characteristics of restless legs syndrome: a study of 133 patients diagnosed with new standard criteria. *Mov Disord.* 1997;12:61-65.

42. Winkelmann J, Wetter TC, Collado-Seidel V, et al. Clinical characteristics and frequency of the hereditary restless legs syndrome in a population of 300 patients. *Sleep.* 2000;23:597-602.

43. Phillips B, Hening W, Britz P, et al. Prevalence and correlates of restless legs syndrome: results from the 2005 National Sleep Foundation Poll. *Chest.* 2006;129:76-80.

44. Michaud M, Soucy JP, Chabli A, Lavigne G, Montplasir J. SPECT imaging of striatal pre- and postsynaptic dopaminergic status in restless legs syndrome with periodic limb movements in sleep. *J Neurol.* 2002;249:164-170.

45. Earley CJ, Connor JR, Beard JL, Malecki EA, Epstein DK, Allen RP. Abnormalities in CSF concentrations of ferritin and transferrin in restless legs syndrome. *Neurology.* 2000;54:1698-1700.

46. Trenkwalder C, Hening WA, Walters AS, Campbell SS, Rahman K, Chokroverty S. Circadian rhythm of periodic limb movements and sensory symptoms of restless legs syndrome. *Mov Disord.* 1999;14:102-110.

47. Allen RP, Barker PB, Wehrl F, Song HK, Earley CJ. MRI measurement of brain iron in patients with restless legs syndrome. *Neurology.* 2001;56:263-265.

48. Connor JR, Boyer PJ, Menzies SL, et al. Neuropathological examination suggests impaired brain iron acquisition in restless legs syndrome. *Neurology.* 2003;61:304-309.

49. Silber MH, Richardson JW. Multiple blood donations associated with iron deficiency in patients with restless legs syndrome. *Mayo Clin Proc.* 2003;78:52-54.

50. International Restless Legs Syndrome Study Group. Validation of the International Restless Legs Syndrome Study Group rating scale for restless legs syndrome. *Sleep Med.* 2003;4:121-132.

51. Allen RP, Becker P, Bogan R, et al. Restless legs syndrome: The efficacy of ropinirole in the treatment of RLS patients suffering from periodic leg movements of sleep. *Sleep.* 2003;26(suppl):A341.

5

52. The International Classification of Sleep Disorders. *Diagnositic and Coding Manual*. 2nd ed. Westchester, Ill; American Academy of Sleep Medicine; 2005.

53. Doghramji K, Browman CP, Gaddy JR, Walsh JK. Triazolam diminishes daytime sleepiness and sleep fragmentation in patients with periodic leg movements in sleep. *J Clin Psychopharmacol.* 1991;11:284-290.

54. Skene DJ, Lockley SW, Arendt J. Use of melatonin in the treatment of phase shift and sleep disorders. *Adv Exp Med Biol.* 1999;467:79-84.

55. Provigil [package insert]. West Chester, Pa: Cephalon, Inc; 2004.

56. Sack RL, Brandes RW, Kendall AR, et al. Entrainment of free-running circadian rhythms by melatonin in blind people. *N Engl J Med.* 2000;343:1070-1077.

57. Leger D, Guilleminault C, Defrance R, et al. Prevalence of sleep/wake disorders in persons with blindness. *Clin Sci (Lond).* 1999;97:193-199.

58. Leger D, Guilleminault C, Santos C, et al. Sleep/wake cycles in the dark: sleep recorded by polysomnography in 26 totally blind subjects compared to controls. *Clin Neurophysiol.* 2002;113:1607-1614.

59. Fischer S, Smolnik R, Herms M, et al. Melatonin acutely improves the neuroendocrine architecture of sleep in blind individuals. *J Clin Endocrinol Metab.* 2003;88:5315-5320.

60. Hack LM, Lockley SW, Arendt J, et al. The effects of low-dose 0.5-mg melatonin on the free-running circadian rhythms of blind subjects. *J Biol Rhythms.* 2003;18:420-429.

61. Mistlberger RE, Skene DJ. Nonphotic entrainment in humans? *J Biol Rhythms.* 2005;20:339-352.

6

Evaluation and Diagnosis

Evaluation of the patient with insomnia begins with a high index of suspicion for its occurrence. Paradoxically, even though it is a prevalent problem that is quite disturbing to patients, it is not often brought to the attention of the clinician. In one study, only 6% of chronic insomniacs seeking medical attention presented primarily for the sleep problem; 25% of patients brought it up as a secondary issue, while the remaining 70% never mentioned it at all.[1] Interestingly, in one study, patients who initiated discussions regarding insomnia with their physicians were those who had experienced insomnia longer, felt worse physically, were older, and were of higher income.[2] Other countries have shown similar trends of patients avoiding insomnia discussions, citing insomnia as being merely an inconvenience.[3]

It should be noted that physicians' tendency to look for this "hidden" problem is low. Barriers to actively seeking out the insomniac are many.[4] Evidence from epidemiologic studies, physician surveys, and clinical studies suggest that several factors contribute to the fact that insomnia is largely unrecognized and inadequately treated, including inadequate physician training in insomnia, belief that sleep complaints are not important; perception that treatments for insomnia are ineffective or associated with risks, and lack of evidence that treating insomnia improves outcomes of comorbid conditions.[4,5] Physician barriers in particular include the perception that sleep problems are less important than other complaints, time limitations during inappropriately abbreviated office visits, Food and Drug Administration labeling and insurance coverage adhering to outdated National Institutes of Health recommendations with restrictions in prescribing, and lack of outcome data addressing whether insomnia management improves either morbidity or mortality.[6]

Clearly, when all the consequences of and associations with insomnia are taken into consideration, and with it being such a ubiquitous problem, the clinician's sense of urgency should rise in looking for the valuable clue in a sleep disturbance. Every office consultation provides an opportunity not only to diagnose insomnia in patients presenting with sleep complaints but also in those with coexistent illnesses and seemingly unrelated symptoms.

Some *acute visit* chief complaints prompting questioning regarding sleep include:

- Statements such as:
  - I'm tired all the time... I have no pep... no energy
  - I don't feel like myself
  - I feel keyed up
  - I'm stressed out
- Chronic sore throat
- Chronic daily headache, especially upon awakening
- Chronic pain
- Chronic cough
- Shortness of breath
- Drug or alcohol abuse
- Urinary frequency/urgency
- Menstrual irregularities, as well as menopause
- Memory problems.

Some *regularly scheduled visit* problems prompting questions regarding sleep include:

- Chronic pain
- Psychiatric problems
- Substance abuse

- Obesity
- Primary sleep disorders
- Neurologic problems such as:
  - Alzheimer's disease
  - Parkinson's disease
  - Peripheral neuropathy
  - Chronic daily headache
  - Migraine headache
- Heart disease, angina, or moderate to severe congestive heart failure (CHF)
- Respiratory disease, especially chronic obstructive pulmonary disease (COPD) or asthma
- Gastrointestinal diseases, such as chronic gastroesophageal reflux disease or irritable bowel syndrome
- Endocrine problems:
  - Perimenopausal
  - Diabetes mellitus
  - Thyroid disease
- Systemic cancer
- Urologic conditions, such as overactive bladder or benign prostatic hyperplasia.

During a comprehensive physical evaluation, there are many aspects that raise the index of suspicion for insomnia (**Table 3.1**) while one is taking the patient's health inventory. Whether prompted by chief complaint, history of present illness, past medical/surgical/psychiatric history, medication list, family history, and social history, the review of systems should also include sleep-related questions.

The main tool in detecting the presence of sleep disturbance is the patient interview, with substantial benefit added by input from the bed partner.[7] The first two questions should be regarding the details of sleep:

- Do you have trouble falling or staying asleep?
- Is your sleep fully refreshing?

Follow-up questions should obtain the details:

- What time do you go to bed?
- How long does it take for you to fall asleep?
- What (if anything) prevents your falling asleep?
- Do you wake up in the middle of the night? What prevents your staying asleep?
- What time do you wake up? Is this normal for you?
- How long has this been occurring?
- What were your sleep patterns like when you were sleeping well?
- How often does the sleep problem occur?
- Has it occurred before? And if so, what did you do about it?
- Does anyone in your immediate family have a similar problem?
- What, if anything, troubles you about your sleep problem?

Consequently, questions regarding daytime issues associated with insomnia should follow:

- How is your energy during the day?
- Do you feel sleepy or nod off when you are idle?
- What do *you* think your sleep problem is causing during the day?
  - Are you having problems functioning at home, work, or social settings?
  - Ask specifically regarding diminished motivation and cognitive dysfunction, such as reduced concentration, vigilance, and memory disruption.

It is also appropriate to ask questions regarding the patient's sleep hygiene:

- Is your bedroom "sleep friendly" (quiet, safe, comfortable, dark)?
- Do you do anything in bed other than sleep and intimate activities?

- Do you eat a large meal at night, and is your supper within 3 hours of bedtime?
- Do you exercise within 4 hours of bedtime?
- Do you smoke too close to bedtime?
- Do you drink alcohol at night? Is it done to help you to go to sleep?
- Do you find yourself staring at the alarm clock, worried about your sleep?

Self-administered questionnaires have also been developed; advantages include saving time for the clinician, allowing more time for the patient to reflect on the questions, and making the questionnaire a permanent part of the patient's record. An example of a sleep hygiene questionnaire for patients is shown in **Figure 6.1**.[8] The Pittsburgh Sleep Quality Index, which provides information about sleep quality, timing, and duration, is shown in **Figure 6.2**.[9]

Certain comorbid insomnia and sleep-related problems can result in or coincide with daytime sleepiness, most notably obstructive sleep apnea syndrome (OSAS), restless legs syndrome (RLS), chronic pain, medications, dementia, shift-work sleep disorder, and depression. In these instances, it may be useful and prudent to quantify the degree of daytime impairment using the Epworth Sleepiness Scale (**Figure 6.3**).[10] This validated instrument also has benefits in displaying to patients in number form the degree of their sleepiness, as well as showing progress during the treatment phase with repeated administration over time.[10]

It should be emphasized that when sleep-related issues are pursued, the following items should be obtained or updated, with specific attention to association with sleep problems:
- Medical history
- Medication list

FIGURE 6.1 — Sleep Hygiene Self-Test Questionnaire

On three or more occasions in the past month, have you:	Yes	No
1. Stretched your muscles (eg, arms, back, legs) regularly during the day?		
2. Drunk coffee, tea, cocoa, or colas or other caffeinated soft drinks after noon?		
3. Eaten chocolate candies or desserts (including ice cream) after dinnertime?		
4. Taken pain relievers that contain caffeine or other stimulants?		
5. Taken any stimulants or over-the-counter "stay alert" pills?		
6. Walked rather than driven to work, to the store, to visit friends, and so on?		
7. Taken any over-the-counter diet pills?		
8. Missed meals or eaten main meals at widely varying times?		
9. Eaten dinner within 2 hours of bedtime?		
10. Eaten spicy foods or snacks within 2 hours before bedtime?		
11. Followed a formal exercise program and exercised?		
12. Drunk 12 oz or more of water, soda, and so on, within 1 hour before bedtime?		
13. Drunk alcohol or alcohol-based sleep medication to help you get to sleep?		
14. Exercised rigorously within 2 hours before bedtime?		
15. Slept late into the morning (more than 90 minutes after usual waking time)?		
16. Gone to bed at roughly the same time?		

17. Watched television up until bedtime?			
18. Talked on the phone for long periods within 2 hours before bedtime?			
19. Taken naps during the day?			
20. Eaten meals or snacks in your bed?			
21. Engaged in daily activities during which your heart rate increased significantly?			
22. Tossed and turned for hours in your bed?			
23. Gotten up in the middle of the night and had a cigarette?			
24. Fallen asleep with the television, radio, or stereo turned on?			
25. Slept in a room that was uncomfortably hot or cold?			
26. Relaxed by reading, listening to soothing music, and so on before going to bed?			
27. Slept with the light on or a light shining into your bedroom?			
28. Slept in a room where you were bothered by noises of some sort?			
29. Awakened in the middle of the night and drunk cola, alcohol, tea, or coffee?			
30. Awakened in the night and tried to make sense of a dream or nightmare?			
Total Score			

For questions 1, 6, 11, 16, 21, and 26, "yes" is scored as 0 and "no" is scored as 1. For all other questions, "yes" is scored as 1 and "no" is scored as 0. Lower total scores indicate more adaptive sleep hygiene.

Blake DD, et al. *Psychol Rep*. 1998;83:1175-1178.

6

FIGURE 6.2 — Pittsburgh Sleep Quality Index (PSQI)

Instructions: The following questions relate to your usual sleep habits during the past month only. Your answers should indicate the most accurate reply for the majority of days and nights in the past month. Please answer all questions.

During the past month:

1. When have you usually gone to bed? ....
2. How long (in minutes) has it taken you to fall asleep each night? ....
3. When have you usually gotten up in the morning? ....
4. How many hours of actual sleep did you get that night (this may be different than the number of hours you spent in bed)?

5. How often have you had trouble sleeping because you:	Not during the past month (0)	Less than once a week (1)	Once or twice a week (2)	Three or more times a week (3)
a. Cannot get to sleep within 30 minutes.	___	___	___	___
b. Wake up in the middle of the night or early morning	___	___	___	___
c. Have to get up to use the bathroom.	___	___	___	___
d. Cannot breathe comfortably.	___	___	___	___
e. Cough or snore loudly	___	___	___	___
f. Feel too cold	___	___	___	___
g. Feel too hot	___	___	___	___
h. Have bad dreams.	___	___	___	___
i. Have pain.	___	___	___	___

j. Other reason(s), please describe, including how often ..... _____
you have had trouble sleeping because of this reason(s): _____

	Very Good (0)	Fairly Good (1)	Fairly Bad (2)	Very Bad (3)
6. How often have you taken medicine (prescribed or over-the-counter) to help you sleep?	—	—	—	—
7. How often have you had trouble staying awake while driving, eating meals, or engaging in social activity?	—	—	—	—
8. How much of a problem has it been for you to keep up enthusiasm to get things done?	—	—	—	—
9. How would you rate your sleep quality overall?	—	—	—	—

Component 1   #9 Score: .... C1 _____

Component 2   #2 Score: (≤15 min = 0, 16-30 min = 1, 31-60 min = 2, >60 min = 3) ...... C2 _____
+ #5a. Score (if sum is equal to 0 = 0, 1-2 = 1, 3-4 = 2, 5-6 = 3)

Component 3   #4 Score (>7 = 0, 6-7 = 1, 5-6 = 2, <5 = 3) .... C3 _____

Component 4   (Total # of hours asleep/total # of hours in bed) × 100. .... C4 _____
(>85% = 0, 75%-84% = 1, 65%-74% = 2, <65% = 3)

Component 5   #5 Score: sum of scores 5b to 5j (0 = 0, 1-0 = 1, 10-28 = 2, 19-27 = 3) ... C5 _____

Component 6   #6 Score. .... C6 _____

Component 7   #7 Score + #8 score (0 = 0, 1-2 = 1, 3-4 = 2, 5-6 = 3) .... C7 _____

Add the seven components scores together _____   Global PSQI Score _____

6

FIGURE 6.3 — Epworth Sleepiness Scale

Situation	Chance of Dozing (0-3)			
Sitting and reading	0	1	2	3
Watching television	0	1	2	3
Sitting inactive in a public place (for example, a theater or meeting)	0	1	2	3
As a passenger in a car for an hour without a break	0	1	2	3
Lying down to rest in the afternoon	0	1	2	3
Sitting and talking to someone	0	1	2	3
Sitting quietly after lunch (when you've had no alcohol)	0	1	2	3
In a car, while stopped in traffic	0	1	2	3
Total Score				

Score Key: 0 = would never doze; 1 = slight chance of dozing; 2 = moderate chance of dozing; 3 = high chance of dosing.

Epworth Sleepiness Scale (ESS) total score ≥10 indicates possible excessive sleepiness or sleep disorder.

Johns MW. *Sleep.* 1991;14:540-545.

- Drug/alcohol/tobacco use
- Family history.

At this point, the information about the individual, coupled with the sleep inventory just gathered, will often clarify the etiology or association of the sleep problem. Physical and psychiatric examinations are differential driven and individual based. The usual minimum examination includes:

- Vital signs, body mass index:
  - Look for resistant hypertension
- Head, eyes, ears, nose, and throat:
  - Look for nasal obstruction (polyps, septal deviation)
  - Look for airway obstruction ("crowded" pharynx,[11] micrognathia)
  - Conjunctival color
- Neck:
  - Look for thyromegaly, nodules, jugular venous distention, carotid pulses
  - Size: >17" in men and >16" in women correlates higher with OSAS[12]
- Heart:
  - CHF
- Lung
  - Asthma
  - COPD
- Extremities:
  - Edema
  - Pulses.

A comprehensive approach to the evaluation of a patient with insomnia is outlined in **Table 6.1**.[13]

It should be noted that the pursuit of knowledge about sleep-related problems usually requires extra time, clinical acumen, interview skills, and especially more information than usual problems. For this reason

TABLE 6.1 — Evaluation of the Patient With Insomnia

State of Assessment	Goal	What to Look For
Initial screening	Identify the nature of the sleep complaint	• Is there difficulty initiating or maintaining sleep? • Experience early awakenings? • Is sleep nonrestorative?
	Determine presence of daytime consequences	• Daytime consequences are required for a diagnosis of insomnia
	Determine the frequency of the complaint	• Chronic insomnia: 2-3 nights/week
	Duration	• ≥1 Month suggests subacute or chronic insomnia
Additional history: precipitating factors, course, and progression of the disease	Factors that alleviate or exacerbate the complaint	• Is the complaint worsened by stress or medical/psychological factors? • Is it easier to sleep away from home or when not trying to sleep? • Is there a conditioned arousal in response to trying to sleep?
	Sleep-wake schedule	• Information from sleep log: Is there evidence for phase advance or delay or irregular patterns? • Does the patient do shift work?

Other nocturnal symptoms or events		• Nightmares, terror, panic, parasomnia (and other behavioral), headache, pain, reflux, nocturia, night sweats, hot flashes, sleep paralysis, hallucinations
	Associated behaviors	• Physical, emotional, or cognitive overactivity before sleep; nocturnal waking behaviors (prolonged time in bed without sleep); food or substance ingestion just prior to sleep
	Sleep-related thoughts	• Negative expectations ("I'll never be able to sleep") • Distortions—erroneous assumptions about sleep needs • Creating catastrophic scenarios around sleep loss
Assess for precipitating or causative factors		• Psychiatric disorders: mood, anxiety, or other psychiatric disorders • Substance misuse or medication use: bronchodilators, steroids, diuretics, stimulants, antihypertensives, activating antidepressants, hypnotic rebound • Medical/neurologic illness: chronic pain, nocturnal headache, gastroesophageal reflux disease, chronic lung disease, nocturnal angina, congestive heart failure, end-stage renal disease, cancer, HIV/AIDS, menopause, dementias, stroke • Sleep disorders: OSA, PLMD, and other movement disorders
Previous treatments: responses and attitudes		

Abbreviations: AIDS, acquired imunodeficiency syndrome; HIV, human immunodeficiency virus; OSA, obstructive sleep apnea; PLMD, periodic limb movement disorder.

Adapted from: Sateia MJ, et al. *Lancet*. 2004;364:1959-1973.

6

and since patients often leave sleep-related symptoms as a "doorknob" complaint (mention it as the clinician has completed the visit and is leaving), it is often appropriate to continue gathering more data at another office visit, as well as to ask the patient to keep a sleep diary or log.[14] Patients may not have been attuned to some subtleties of their sleep characteristics, like sleep latency, duration of time awake if awakened, daytime distress, etc. One example of a sleep log is shown in **Figure 6.4**. Other diaries are also available online, one being interactive by the National Sleep Foundation (http://www.sleepfoundation.org/quiz/index.php?secid+&id=107).

Laboratory testing is also differential driven. For example, the patient with presumed RLS should have blood chemistries to rule out secondary causes (see Chapter 5, *Common Conditions Associated With Insomnia*). Obtaining a chemistry panel, complete blood count, and thyroid-stimulating hormone test may be fruitful in allaying fears about an internal problem and allow the patient to more eagerly pursue the course deemed appropriate by the clinician.

Referral for sleep testing can be accomplished with or without consultation with a sleep specialist. However, in some instances, the option of a direct referral by the primary care physician to the sleep laboratory is not available. A consultation with a sleep specialist then becomes necessary, causing a delay in testing. However, in certain cases, such a consultation is warranted. Examples include the need for testing that is more complex and extensive than the standard overnight polysomnogram (extended EEG leads for detection of nocturnal epilepsy, addition of daytime maintenance of wakefulness testing, etc) and cases of chronic insomnia that do not require testing but for which the input from a sleep specialist might be helpful. Appropriate instances in which either sleep consultation and/or testing is warranted include[14-16]:

- Suspected sleep disorder
  - Obstructive sleep apnea
  - Narcolepsy
  - Periodic limb movement disorder
- Unexplained sleepiness/tiredness
- Unusual parasomnias
  - Violent behavior while sleeping
- Treatment issues
  - Insomnia and sleep problems resistant to treatment.

REFERENCES

1. Ancoli-Israel S, Roth T. Characteristics of insomnia in the United States: results of the 1991 National Sleep Foundation Survey. I. *Sleep*. 1999;22(suppl 2):S347-S353.

2. Shochat T, Umphress J, Israel AG, Ancoli-Israel S. Insomnia in primary care patients. *Sleep*. 1999;22(suppl 2):S359-S365.

3. Terzano MG, Parrino L, Cirignotta F, et al; Studio Morfeo Committee. Studio Morfeo: insomnia in primary care, a survey conducted on the Italian population. *Sleep Med*. 2004;5:67-75.

4. Benca RM. Diagnosis and treatment of chronic insomnia: a review. *Psychiatr Serv*. 2005;56:332-343.

5. Winkelman JW. A Primary Care Approach to Insomnia Management. Medscape, 2005. Available at: http://www.medscape.com/viewprogram/3807. Accessed on December 13, 2006.

6. Israel AG, Lieberman JA. Tackling insomnia: diagnostic and treatment issues in primary care. In: *Insomnia in Primary Care. Postgraduate Medicine Special Report*. 2004;7-13.

7. Kupfer DJ, Reynolds CF 3rd. Management of insomnia. *N Engl J Med*. 1997;336:341-346.

8. Blake DD, Gomez MH. A scale for assessing sleep hygiene: preliminary data. *Psychol Rep*. 1998;83:1175-1178.

9. Buysse DJ, Reynolds CF 3rd, Monk TH, Berman SR, Kupfer DJ. The Pittsburgh Sleep Quality Index: a new instrument for psychiatric practice and research. *Psychiatry Res*. 1989;28:193-213.

FIGURE 6.4 — Personal Sleep Diary

	Day 1 Date	Day 2 Date	Day 3 Date	Day 4 Date	Day 5 Date	Day 6 Date	Day 7 Date
Time I went to bed last night	___ AM ___ PM	___ AM ___ PM	___ AM ___ PM	___ AM ___ PM	___ AM ___ PM	___ AM ___ PM	___ AM ___ PM
Time I woke this morning	___ AM	___ AM	___ AM	___ AM	___ AM	___ AM	___ AM
Time it took to fall asleep last night	___ minutes	___ minutes	___ minutes	___ minutes	___ minutes	___ minutes	___ minutes
Sleep duration last night	___ hours	___ hours	___ hours	___ hours	___ hours	___ hours	___ hours
Number of awakenings and total time awake last night	___ minutes	___ minutes	___ minutes	___ minutes	___ minutes	___ minutes	___ minutes
Causes of sleep disturbance(s) last night (list any mental, emotional, physical, or environmental factors that affected sleep)	___ ___ ___	___ ___ ___	___ ___ ___	___ ___ ___	___ ___ ___	___ ___ ___	___ ___ ___
I would rate the quality of my sleep last night as being	☐ Poor ☐ Fair ☐ Good ☐ Excellent	☐ Poor ☐ Fair ☐ Good ☐ Excellent	☐ Poor ☐ Fair ☐ Good ☐ Excellent	☐ Poor ☐ Fair ☐ Good ☐ Excellent	☐ Poor ☐ Fair ☐ Good ☐ Excellent	☐ Poor ☐ Fair ☐ Good ☐ Excellent	☐ Poor ☐ Fair ☐ Good ☐ Excellent
I feel that I had an adequate amount of sleep last night	☐ Yes ☐ No	☐ Yes ☐ No	☐ Yes ☐ No	☐ Yes ☐ No	☐ Yes ☐ No	☐ Yes ☐ No	☐ Yes ☐ No
How awake did I feel when I got up this morning	☐ Wide awake ☐ Awake but a little tired ☐ Sleepy	☐ Wide awake ☐ Awake but a little tired ☐ Sleepy	☐ Wide awake ☐ Awake but a little tired ☐ Sleepy	☐ Wide awake ☐ Awake but a little tired ☐ Sleepy	☐ Wide awake ☐ Awake but a little tired ☐ Sleepy	☐ Wide awake ☐ Awake but a little tired ☐ Sleepy	☐ Wide awake ☐ Awake but a little tired ☐ Sleepy

Complete in the Morning

I was sleepy during the day today	☐ Yes ☐ No	☐ Yes ☐ No	☐ Yes ☐ No	☐ Yes ☐ No	☐ Yes ☐ No	☐ Yes ☐ No	☐ Yes ☐ No
Number of caffeinated drinks (coffee, tea, cola) and time drank	___ AM/PM	___ AM/PM	___ AM/PM	___ AM/PM	___ AM/PM	___ AM/PM	___ AM/PM
Number of alcoholic drinks (beer, wine, liquor) and time drank	___ AM/PM	___ AM/PM	___ AM/PM	___ AM/PM	___ AM/PM	___ AM/PM	___ AM/PM
I took a nap today (list time taken and duration)	___ AM/PM ___ minutes	___ AM/PM ___ minutes	___ AM/PM ___ minutes	___ AM/PM ___ minutes	___ AM/PM ___ minutes	___ AM/PM ___ minutes	___ AM/PM ___ minutes
I exercised at least 20 minutes today	☐ No ☐ Morning ☐ Afternoon ☐ Within 2-3 hours of retiring	☐ No ☐ Morning ☐ Afternoon ☐ Within 2-3 hours of retiring	☐ No ☐ Morning ☐ Afternoon ☐ Within 2-3 hours of retiring	☐ No ☐ Morning ☐ Afternoon ☐ Within 2-3 hours of retiring	☐ No ☐ Morning ☐ Afternoon ☐ Within 2-3 hours of retiring	☐ No ☐ Morning ☐ Afternoon ☐ Within 2-3 hours of retiring	☐ No ☐ Morning ☐ Afternoon ☐ Within 2-3 hours of retiring
Complete in the Evening							
I consumed nicotine after 6:00 p.m.	☐ Yes ☐ No	☐ Yes ☐ No	☐ Yes ☐ No	☐ Yes ☐ No	☐ Yes ☐ No	☐ Yes ☐ No	☐ Yes ☐ No
I consumed a heavy meal or snack after 6:00 PM	☐ Yes ☐ No	☐ Yes ☐ No	☐ Yes ☐ No	☐ Yes ☐ No	☐ Yes ☐ No	☐ Yes ☐ No	☐ Yes ☐ No
About 1 hour before going to sleep, I did the following activity (list activity, eg. watch TV, work, read)							
Medications taken before retiring, amount, and time taken	___ PM	___ PM	___ PM	___ PM	___ PM	___ PM	___ PM

6

10. Johns MW. A new method for measuring daytime sleepiness: the Epworth sleepiness scale. *Sleep.* 1991;14:540-545.

11. Lam B, Ip MS, Tench E, Ryan CF. Craniofacial profile in Asian and white subjects with obstructive sleep apnoea. *Thorax.* 2005;60:504-510.

12. Dancey DR, Hanly PJ, Soong C, Lee B, Shepard J Jr, Hoffstein V. Gender differences in sleep apnea: the role of neck circumference. *Chest.* 2003;123:1544-1550.

13. Sateia MJ, Nowell PD. Insomnia. *Lancet.* 2004;364:1959-1973.

14. Sateia MJ, Doghramji K, Hauri PJ, Morin CM. Evaluation of chronic insomnia. An American Academy of Sleep Medicine review. *Sleep.* 2000;23:243-308.

15. Doghramji PP. Detection of insomnia in primary care. *J Clin Psychiatry.* 2001;62(suppl 10):18-26.

16. Kushida CA, Littner MR, Morgenthaler T, et al. Practice parameters for the indications for polysomnography and related procedures: an update for 2005. *Sleep.* 2005;28:499-521.

7

Management: General Considerations and Comorbid Insomnia

Symptom or Syndrome?

As discussed in Chapter 3, *Insomnia: Definition, Diagnostic Terms, Demographics, and Impairments*, insomnia is classified into four categories: [1]

- Primary insomnia
- Related to a mental disorder
- Due to a general medical condition
- Substance induced.

Primary insomnia, by definition, is a sleep problem with no identifiable cause or comorbidities, while the latter three may have specific causes or comorbidities. In other words, insomnia, like pain, may be a symptom of or comorbid with another medical or psychological disorder, or it may be a syndrome in and of itself. Since primary insomnia is seen in only approximately 10% to 20% of patients with sleep problems in a primary care setting, diagnosis and treatment of sleep disorders of necessity require comprehensive evaluation of the patient's medical, psychological, and social status. **Figure 7.1** illustrates a practical algorithm for the evaluation and treatment of patients who present with sleep disorders.[2]

When and How Soon to Treat Comorbid Insomnia

Since insomnia is most commonly a symptom of or comorbid with some other medical or psychiatric

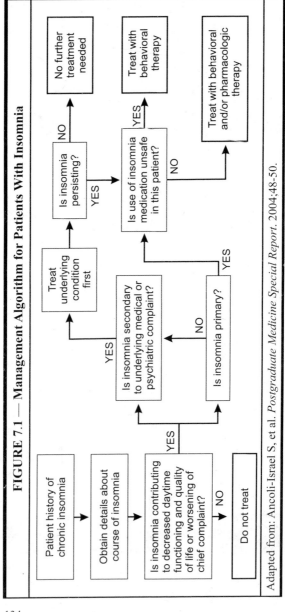

FIGURE 7.1 — Management Algorithm for Patients With Insomnia

Patient history of chronic insomnia → Obtain details about course of insomnia → Is insomnia contributing to decreased daytime functioning and quality of life or worsening of chief complaint?

NO → Do not treat

YES → Is insomnia secondary to underlying medical or psychiatric complaint?

Is insomnia primary?

NO → Is insomnia primary?

YES (insomnia secondary) → Treat underlying condition first → Is insomnia persisting?

NO → No further treatment needed

YES → Is use of insomnia medication unsafe in this patient?

YES → Treat with behavioral therapy

NO → Treat with behavioral and/or pharmacologic therapy

Adapted from: Ancoli-Israel S, et al. *Postgraduate Medicine Special Report.* 2004;48-50.

condition, an important question facing the clinician is whether specific treatment of the insomnia should be delayed until the underlying cause or comorbidity is identified and treated, or whether it should be managed at the outset. In most cases, there are several reasons for not waiting to treat the insomnia.

First, one obvious and important reason for not waiting is that since the identification and/or successful treatment of the cause or comorbidity may take time, the patient's sleep problems may continue to cause significant distress and possibly daytime dysfunction. Thus alleviating difficulty in sleeping may not only relieve an uncomfortable symptom but also improve quality of life. This is analogous to reducing pain while the cause of the pain is under investigation.

Second, the patient's sleep problems may not have an underlying cause or association with other conditions. Primary insomnia may coexist with, yet not be caused by, other conditions. In these instances, the choice of treatment given to patients can be made at the time of diagnosis, as well as instituting treatment of the coexisting condition at that time.

Third, data are emerging to suggest that symptomatic management of the insomnia can benefit the comorbid condition itself. For example, as discussed below, in patients with major depressive disorder (MDD) and insomnia, concurrent treatment of insomnia and depression has resulted in better outcomes than treating the depression alone.

■ **Insomnia and Major Depressive Disorder**

In patients with comorbid insomnia and MDD, three general treatment strategies apply:
- Monotherapy: Treatment of the MDD and coexisting insomnia with an antidepressant alone
- Polytherapy: Antidepressant for MDD and sedating agent for insomnia

- Nonpharmacologic techniques: Although these methods have not been extensively examined in the context of MDD with coexisting insomnia, there is ample evidence that they are highly effective for the treatment of primary insomnia and MDD. Nonpharmacologic techniques for the treatment of primary insomnia are reviewed in Chapter 8, *Behavioral Strategies and Nonprescription Agents*.

Monotherapy

The effects of antidepressants on polysomnographic sleep patterns have been extensively reviewed.[3] However, these effects may not yet have direct clinical relevance for the primary care physician and are of greater research interest than clinical interest. Regarding their subjective effects, which may be of greater clinical relevance, studies indicate that antidepressants, when administered at doses appropriate for the treatment of depression (as opposed to low-dose strategies) are effective in decreasing sleep complaints in depressed patients when they are considered as a group.[4]

However, individual patients may also experience either nonimprovement or even a worsening of insomnia complaints. Studies reveal that nearly half of patients meeting criteria for a full response for depression have a persistent difficulty with sleep (**Figure 7.2**).[5] The reasons for these negative effects are difficult to discern in any given case. However, they may be due to:

- Poor response of the underlying depression to that particular antidepressant; the persistent insomnia can represent evidence of a persistent depression, in which case additional time on antidepressant medication, increasing the dosage, augmenting it with another antidepres-

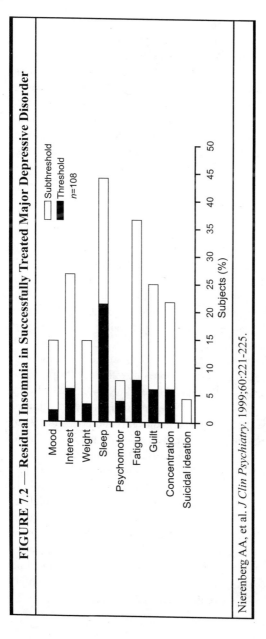

FIGURE 7.2 — Residual Insomnia in Successfully Treated Major Depressive Disorder

Nierenberg AA, et al. *J Clin Psychiatry.* 1999;60:221-225.

sant, or switching the antidepressant agent should be considered.

- Iatrogenic effect of the antidepressant medication, ie, disruptive effect on sleep, in which case additional time on antidepressant medication may impart some degree of tolerance to these effects. Additional measures include decreasing the dosage of the antidepressant medication, yet this may be a poor strategy since it risks the possibility of diminishing its effect against depression. Another option would be to utilize the polytherapy options (discussed later).

Prior to instituting treatment with an antidepressant, it would be beneficial to have available a profile of the various antidepressants regarding their relative effects on sleep. Unfortunately, very little research has been done in directly comparing the sleep effects of antidepressants with one another. In one of the largest studies in this area, an 8-week comparison between fluoxetine and nefazodone in MDD patients indicated that both antidepressants diminished sleep-related complaints, yet nefazodone was superior to fluoxetine for sleep-related complaints at the end of 8 weeks, despite equal efficacy for depression (**Figure 7.3**).[6-8] This study was limited by the lack of a placebo-control condition. The use of nefazodone, however, has fallen dramatically due to reports of its association with liver failure.

Based on individual, noncomparative studies, antidepressants that have sedating effects include several tricyclic antidepressants (TCAs) (amitriptyline, imipramine, doxepin, and trimipramine), trazodone, nefazodone, and mirtazapine. Those that may be more disruptive of sleep include nonsedating TCAs (clomipramine, desipramine, and protriptyline), monoamine oxidase inhibitors, selective serotonin reuptake inhibitors (SSRIs), venlafaxine, and bupropion.[9]

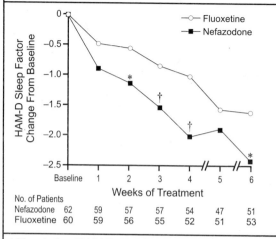

FIGURE 7.3 — Nefazodone vs Fluoxetine Subjective Sleep

No. of Patients	Baseline	1	2	3	4	5	6
Nefazodone	62	59	57	57	54	47	51
Fluoxetine	60	59	56	55	52	51	53

Abbreviation: HAM-D, Hamilton Depression [scale].

* *P* <0.05 compared with fluoxetine.
† *P* <0.01 compared with fluoxetine.

Armitage R, et al. *J Clin Psychopharmacol.* 1997;17:161-168; Gillin JC, et al. *J Clin Psychiatry.* 1997;58:185-192; Rush AJ, et al. *Biol Psychiatry.* 1998;44:3-14.

Polytherapy

There is some evidence that the addition of low doses of sedating antidepressants to the already existing antidepressant may have some benefit. The most widely utilized agent for this purpose is trazodone, although it is not, nor is any other antidepressant, approved by the Food and Drug Administration (FDA) for this use (**Figure 7.4**).[10] In general, 65% to 92% of patients have a good hypnotic response, yet patients may experience daytime sedation. Authors have also cautioned regarding the potential for the development of a "serotonin syndrome" when this agent is combined with antidepressants.[11] Additionally, studies of this

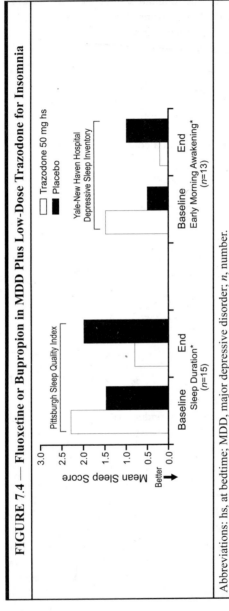

FIGURE 7.4 — Fluoxetine or Bupropion in MDD Plus Low-Dose Trazodone for Insomnia

Abbreviations: hs, at bedtime; MDD, major depressive disorder; *n*, number.

* Significantly more improvement with trazodone than placebo (*P* = 0.005). Change scores greater with trazodone than with placebo (*P* = 0.01).

Adapted from: Nierenberg AA, et al. *Am J Psychiatry*. 1994;151:1069-1072.

use are limited due to small sample sizes and lack of placebo-control conditions. Other agents that have received similar attention in this area are low doses of amitriptyline and doxepin.

Continuing the discussion of the polytherapy option, hypnotic agents have also been examined in the context of MDD patients on antidepressants. Although uncontrolled studies have been performed,[12] only the controlled studies will be reviewed in the discussion that follows. In a controlled, 4-week study of zolpidem 10 mg or placebo at bedtime in SSRI-treated (fluoxetine, sertraline, or paroxetine) MDD patients with persistent insomnia, significant improvement was noted in total sleep time and wake after sleep onset. However, no improvement was noted in depression scores (**Figure 7.5**).[13]

In another study utilizing two hypnotic agents not available in the United States, patients with MDD who were treated with maprotiline or nortriptyline also received either lormetazepam (n=17), flunitrazepam (n=16), or placebo for 4 weeks.[14] As expected, both agents improved sleep. However, of interest in this pilot study was the finding that lormetazepam resulted in a greater decrease in the score on the Hamilton Depression Subscale than placebo ($P = 0.06$), yet this difference only approached statistical significance.

Finally, in a recent randomized, placebo-controlled study, 445 MDD patients with insomnia received 10 weeks of fluoxetine every morning and either eszopiclone 3 mg or placebo nightly for 8 weeks. In addition to significantly improved subjective sleep variables, such as sleep latency, total sleep time, and wake after sleep onset, eszopiclone coadministration resulted in significant reductions in HAM-D scores compared with placebo coadministration. This was seen at week 4, and then with progressive improvement at week 8. To assess the effect of insomnia treatment on depression alone, when HAM-D insomnia items were removed,

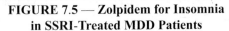

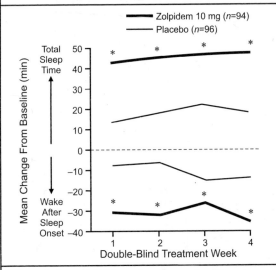

FIGURE 7.5 — Zolpidem for Insomnia in SSRI-Treated MDD Patients

Abbreviations: MDD, major depressive disorder; *n*, number; SSRI, selective serotonin reuptake inhibitor.

* *P* <0.05 vs placebo.

Asnis GM, et al. *J Clin Psychiatry.* 1999;60:668-676.

differences were still seen to be significant at week 8 (*P* <0.03) (**Figure 7.6**).[15] As expected, HAM-D differences were greater in patients with more severe depression. At week 8, significantly more eszopiclone patients were responders (74% vs 61%, *P* <0.009) and remitters (54% vs 41%, *P* <0.02).

The results of these last two studies are of interest in that if confirmed by further studies, they suggest that insomnia itself may be etiologically related to depression in a circular fashion. It should be noted that hypnotics are not FDA indicated for the management of depression.

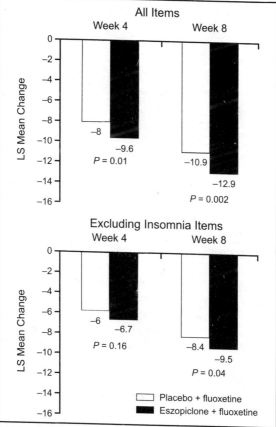

FIGURE 7.6 — Mean Change in 17-Item HAM-D Scores Among All Patients With and Without the Insomnia Items

Abbreviations: HAM-D, Hamilton Depression [scale]; LS, least squares.

P values reflect change from baseline analyses with analysis of covariance.

Fava M, et al. *Biol Psychiatry*. 2006;59:1052-1060.

■ Insomnia and Pain

Pain is another comorbid condition that is bidirectional; not only does it impact sleep, but is itself impacted by sleep problems.[16-18] It is intuitively known that any painful condition will disturb sleep as well as affect mood, energy, cognitive function, and behavior. According to a Gallup Poll Survey, 56 million Americans complain that nighttime pain interferes with their falling asleep and promotes awakenings during the night or early morning.[19] In fact, the greater the pain, the greater the likelihood of insomnia or nonrefreshing sleep.[20] In addition, the sleep problems associated with chronic pain may also be a feature of psychiatric disturbances that occur as a result of physical, psychosocial, vocational, and economic concerns. But as a corollary, if normal, healthy subjects are given several nights of disturbances to the slow-wave (deep) sleep, this has been shown to induce not only nonrefreshing sleep but also nonspecific generalized muscle aching and fatigue.[21-23] Results of other studies have also indicated that the pain-sleep relationship is bidirectional: pain while awake can cause sleeplessness and, in turn, poor-quality sleep can exacerbate pain. This can then cause a vicious circle of increasing pain and sleeplessness, one amplifying the other.[24]

The management of insomnia associated with pain begins by quantifying the sleep disturbance and its consequences, and also the nature of the pain, especially whether it is acute or chronic. Since acute pain causes direct arousals during sleep, consideration should strongly be given to treat pain aggressively with analgesics. But since most pain medications not only cause relief but also have soporific effects, hypnotics are usually not needed. Moreover, there is no evidence that hypnotic medications provide any direct pain-relieving effect.[25] However, in a pilot controlled study of 15 patients, triazolam was found to improve sleep, morning stiffness, and daytime sleepiness in patients with rheumatoid arthritis.[26]

■ Insomnia in Perimenopausal Women

The management of insomnia in perimenopausal women is especially challenging since the prevalence of insomnia rises sharply by approximately 40% during the transition to, through, and after menopause.[27] The evidence for the role of hot flashes in insomnia is mixed since some studies have shown an association between hot flashes and nighttime arousals,[28] while others have not found hot flashes to objectively lessen measures of sleep quality.[29] In addition, sleep disorders are more common at the time of climacteric and may play a role in insomnia during this period. For example, Wisconsin Sleep Cohort data show that menopause is an independent risk factor for obstructive sleep apnea.[30] Depression and anxiety are also more common during this period and must be considered contributory to insomnia.

The management of insomnia in perimenopausal women obviously involves a comprehensive evaluation, since there may be several contributing factors to the insomnia. Hormonal therapy can also be addressed, although use has greatly declined due to evidence of harm with long-term use. In one study, women using hormone replacement therapy were seen to have fewer hot flashes and less insomnia.[31]

Treatment Options

The treatment options for primary and comorbid insomnia are discussed in detail in Chapter 8, *Behavioral Strategies and Nonprescription Agents* and Chapter 9, *Pharmacologic Agents for Insomnia*.

REFERENCES

1. *Diagnostic and Statistical Manual of Psychiatric Disorders.* 4th ed, Text Revision. Washington, DC: American Psychiatric Association; 2000.

2. Ancoli-Israel S, Benca RM, Doghramji PP, et al. Insomnia in primary care. Panel discussion. *Postgraduate Medicine Special Report.* Minneapolis, Minn: McGraw-Hill Medical Information Services; December 2004;48-50.

3. Tsuno N, Besset A, Ritchie K. Sleep and depression. *J Clin Psychiatry.* 2005;66:1254-1269.

4. Satterlee WG, Faries D. The effects of fluoxetine on symptoms of insomnia in depressed patients. *Psychopharmacol Bull.* 1995;31:227-237.

5. Nierenberg AA, Keefe BR, Leslie VC, et al. Residual symptoms in depressed patients who respond acutely to fluoxetine. *J Clin Psychiatry.* 1999;60:221-225.

6. Armitage R, Yonkers K, Cole D, Rush AJ. A multicenter, double-blind comparison of the effects of nefazodone and fluoxetine on sleep architecture and quality of sleep in depressed outpatients. *J Clin Psychopharmacol.* 1997;17:161-168.

7. Gillin JC, Rapaport M, Erman MK, Winokur A, Albala BJ. A comparison of nefazodone and fluoxetine on mood and on objective, subjective, and clinician-rated measures of sleep in depressed patients: a double-blind, 8-week clinical trial. *J Clin Psychiatry.* 1997;58:185-192.

8. Rush AJ, Armitage R, Gillin JC, et al. Comparative effects of nefazodone and fluoxetine on sleep in outpatients with major depressive disorder. *Biol Psychiatry.* 1998;44:3-14.

9. Thase ME. Depression, sleep, and antidepressants. *J Clin Psychiatry.* 1998;59(suppl 4):55-65.

10. Nierenberg AA, Adler LA, Peselow E, Zornberg G, Rosenthal M. Trazodone for antidepressant-associated insomnia. *Am J Psychiatry.* 1994;151:1069-1072.

11. Margolese HC, Chouinard G. Serotonin syndrome from addition of low-dose trazodone to nefazodone. *Am J Psychiatry.* 2000;157:1022.

12. Buysse DJ, Reynolds CF 3rd, Houck PR, et al. Does lorazepam impair the antidepressant response to nortriptyline and psychotherapy? *J Clin Psychiatry*. 1997;58:426-432.

13. Asnis GM, Chakraburtty A, DuBoff EA, et al. Zolpidem for persistent insomnia in SSRI-treated depressed patients. *J Clin Psychiatry*. 1999;60:668-676.

14. Nolen WA, Haffmans PM, Bouvy PF, Duivenvoorden HJ. Hypnotics as concurrent medication in depression. A placebo-controlled, double-blind comparison of flunitrazepam and lormetazepam in patients with major depression, treated with a (tri)cyclic antidepressant. *J Affect Disord*. 1993;28:179-188.

15. Fava M, McCall WV, Krystal A, et al. Eszopiclone co-administered with fluoxetine in patients with insomnia coexisting with major depressive disorder. *Biol Psychiatry*. 2006;59:1052-1060.

16. Cohen MJM, Menefee LA, Doghramji K, Anderson WR, Frank ED. Sleep in chronic pain: problems and treatments. *Int Rev Psychiatry*. 2000;12:115-127.

17. Menefee LA, Frank ED, Doghramji K, et al. Self-reported sleep quality and quality of life for individuals with chronic pain conditions. *Clin J Pain*. 2000;16:290-297.

18. Menefee LA, Cohen MJ, Anderson WR, Doghramji K, Frank ED, Lee H. Sleep disturbance and nonmalignant chronic pain: a comprehensive review of the literature. *Pain Med*. 2000;1:156-172.

19. National Sleep Foundation. Gallup Poll on adult public's experience with nighttime pain. Washington, DC: National Sleep Foundation; 1996:2005.

20. Sutton DA, Moldofsky H, Badley EM. Insomnia and health problems in Canadians. *Sleep*. 2001;24:665-670.

21. Moldofsky H, Scarisbrick P. Induction of neurasthenic musculoskeletal pain syndrome by selective sleep stage deprivation. *Psychosom Med*. 1976;38:35-44.

22. Moldofsky H, Scarisbrick P, England R, Smythe H. Musculo-sketal symptoms and non-REM sleep disturbance in patients with "fibrositis syndrome" and healthy subjects. *Psychosom Med*. 1975;37:341-351.

7

23. Lentz MJ, Landis CA, Rothermel J, Shaver JL. Effects of selective slow wave sleep disruption on musculoskeletal pain and fatigue in middle aged women. *J Rheumatol*. 1999;26:1586-1592.

24. Affleck G, Urrows S, Tennen H, Higgins P, Abeles M. Sequential daily relations of sleep, pain intensity, and attention to pain among women with fibromyalgia. *Pain*. 1996;68:363-368.

25. Jamieson AO. Pain and Sleep. Medscape Primary Care 6, 2004. Posted 08/27/2004. www.medscape.com/viewarticle/487971.

26. Walsh JK, Muehlbach MJ, Lauter SA, Hilliker NA, Schweitzer PK. Effects of triazolam on sleep, daytime sleepiness, and morning stiffness in patients with rheumatoid arthritis. *J Rheumatol*. 1996;23:245-252.

27. Moline ML, Broch L, Zak R. Sleep in women across the life cycle from adulthood through menopause. *Med Clin North Am*. 2004;88:705-736.

28. Freedman RR, Norton D, Woodward S, Cornelissen G. Core body temperature and circadian rhythm of hot flashes in menopausal women. *J Clin Endocrinol Metab*. 1995;80:2354-2358.

29. Polo-Kantola P, Erkkola R, Irjala K, Helenius H, Pullinen S, Polo O. Climacteric symptoms and sleep quality. *Obstet Gynecol*. 1999;94:219-224.

30. Young T, Rabago D, Zgierska A, Austin D, Laurel F. Objective and subjective sleep quality in premenopausal, perimenopausal, and postmenopausal women in the Wisconsin Sleep Cohort Study. *Sleep*. 2003;26:667-672.

31. Owens JF, Matthews KA. Sleep disturbance in healthy middle-aged women. *Maturitas*. 1998;30:41-50.

8

Behavioral Strategies and Nonprescription Agents

Behavioral Strategies

Patients with insomnia can benefit from a range of behavioral interventions, including:

- Sleep hygiene education
- Stimulus control
- Sleep restriction
- Cognitive behavior therapy (CBT)
- Muscle relaxation training
- Biofeedback (most commonly using electromyography)
- Paradoxic intention.

The goals and specific components of these interventions are outlined in **Table 8.1**.[1-5] Although not listed here, bright-light therapy has been shown to be effective in reentrainment of circadian rhythm in patients with sleep-phase disorders (see Chapter 5, *Common Conditions Associated With Insomnia*). These behavioral methods can be used individually or in combinations that typically include sleep hygiene education. Furthermore, these therapies can be delivered in individual treatment settings, in groups, or by means of self-help programs using written materials, tapes, etc.

A number of meta-analyses[4,6,7] reviewed the clinical trial data on many of the behavioral therapies for chronic insomnia and found significant efficacy with large effect sizes for reduction of sleep latency (eg, 0.87–0.88), improvement of sleep quality (eg, 0.94), and moderate effect sizes (eg, 0.49–0.53) for

TABLE 8.1 — Behavioral Strategies for Treating Chronic Insomnia

Sleep Hygiene Education

Goal: To reduce or eliminate maladaptive behaviors
The patient should:
- Maintain a regular sleep-wake schedule; set a regular wake-up time
- Not nap, especially close to bedtime
- Not "sleep in" after a poor night
- Avoid watching the clock
- Avoid alcohol for 4 hours before bedtime
- Avoid caffeine and nicotine for 6 hours before bedtime
- Exercise regularly but avoid strenuous exercise within 3 to 4 hours before bedtime
- Make sure the bedroom is dark and quiet, and that the temperature is comfortable

Stimulus Control

Goal: To remove negative conditioning for sleep
The patient should:
- Go to bed only when sleepy and at a set bedtime
- Get up after 20 minutes if not able to fall asleep or stay asleep
- Return to bed only when feeling sleepy
- Get up at the set wake-up time
- Avoid daytime naps

Sleep Restriction

Goal: To limit time spent in bed to only time spent sleeping
The patient should:
- Maintain a sleep log to determine baseline mean total sleep time
- When sleep time is >90% of baseline, increase sleep time by 15-minute intervals over 5 to 7 days
- When sleep time is <80% of baseline, decrease sleep time by 15-minute intervals over 5 to 7 days
- Repeat time in bed adjustments every 5 to 7 days

Continued

Cognitive Behavior Therapy
Goal: To identify and correct patient misconceptions about sleep *The physician should:* • Correct maladaptive beliefs (eg, "I have a chemical imbalance"; "I can't sleep without medication") • Replace these with realistic/adaptive beliefs

Progressive Muscle Relaxation
Goal: To prepare for sleep by achieving a calm and relaxed state *The patient should:* • In specific order, alternately tense and relax each major muscle group

Biofeedback
Goal: To achieve a calm and relaxed state similar to progressive muscle relaxation most commonly using electromyography (muscle feedback) or less commonly with electroencephalography (eg, theta wave or sleep spindle feedback)

Paradoxic Intention
Goal: To reduce performance anxiety caused by trying to fall asleep *The physician should:* • Encourage the patient to deliberatively attempt to stay awake

Based on information from: Kupfer DJ, et al. *N Engl J Med.* 1997;336:341-346; Sateia MJ, et al. *Lancet.* 2004;364:1959-1973; Benca BM. In: *Insomnia in Primary Care: A Postgraduate Medicine Special Report.* 2004:23-32; Morin CM, et al. *Sleep.* 1999;22:1134-1156; Morin CM. In: *Principles and Practice of Sleep Medicine.* 4th ed. 2005:726-737.

frequency of awaking and total sleep time. Such results suggest that for sleep-onset insomnia, for example, an effect size of 0.87–0.88 means that about 80% of treated patients had significantly shorter sleep latency than controls. In clock time, this meant reductions in sleep latency of 65 minutes compared with

35 minutes among control patients. According to an American Sleep Society Review, between 70% and 80% of patients with chronic insomnia can benefit from behavioral therapy.[4] Another advantage of behavioral treatments for chronic insomnia is that the benefits appear to be sustained for at least 6 months after active treatment has been discontinued.[6]

The American Society of Sleep Medicine Practice guidelines, derived from the above-mentioned meta-analyses as well as individual studies, concluded that stimulus control is the standard for effective treatment, while progressive muscle relaxation and paradoxic intention also meet the criteria for well-validated, effective treatments.[8] Sleep restriction, biofeedback, and multicomponent strategies were considered probably efficacious. Although sleep hygiene education is typically a component of behavioral treatments, it has not been thoroughly studied as an individual intervention.

A recent meta-analysis by Perlis and colleagues[9] compared studies of cognitive and behavioral therapies with others using pharmacotherapy and found that after termination of acute treatment, the two strategies were equally effective, although there were some indications that CBT may be superior for sleep-onset problems. In one study in which CBT, pharmacotherapy, and a combination of the two was used in adults who had chronic sleep-onset insomnia, CBT alone was as effective as CBT in combination with pharmacotherapy (**Figure 8.1**).[10]

In a similar study in elderly patients with chronic primary insomnia, CBT combined with pharmacotherapy was found to be slightly better than with either alone (**Figure 8.2**).[11] Pharmacotherapy benefits appeared early, while it took longer for the benefits of CBT to appear. However, one meta-analysis showed that the benefits of CBT continued long after treatment had stopped, while the benefits of pharmacotherapy ceased as soon as it was withdrawn (**Figure 8.3**).[5]

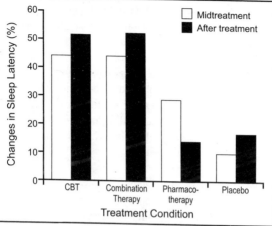

FIGURE 8.1 — CBT and Pharmacotherapy: Changes in Sleep-Onset Latency

Abbreviation: CBT, cognitive behavior therapy.

Jacobs DG, et al. *Arch Intern Med*. 2004;164:1888-1896.

Although behavioral therapy is quite effective and also highly acceptable to patients,[12] it has several limitations. For example, implementation into a primary care or general practice setting requires resources and trained health care professionals to deliver the interventions. Sufficient time must be allotted for each patient, often five to seven sessions, each lasting 30 to 45 minutes, several times per week. There are also patient cost considerations due to restrictive insurance coverage and/or the patient's financial situation. Effective implementation of CBT programs also would require that either the physician or other staff member/office personnel be trained to administer this therapy; currently, such training is not readily available. Finally, patients must be motivated to attend the sessions and adhere to the regimen.

Although no easy solution exists, some evidence suggests that routine incorporation of behavioral thera-

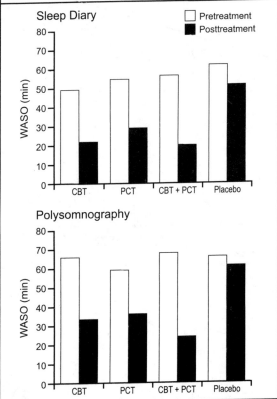

FIGURE 8.2 — Combined Behavioral and Pharmacologic Approaches

Abbreviations: CBT, cognitive behavior therapy; PCT, pharmacotherapy; WASO, wake after sleep onset.

Morin CM, et al. *JAMA*. 1999;281:991-999.

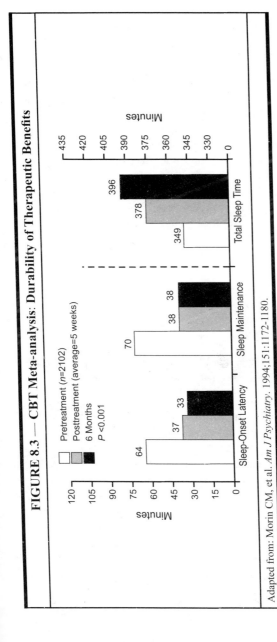

FIGURE 8.3 — CBT Meta-analysis: Durability of Therapeutic Benefits

Pretreatment (*n*=2102)
Posttreatment (average=5 weeks)
6 Months
P <0.001

Sleep-Onset Latency: 64, 37, 33

Sleep Maintenance: 70, 38, 38

Total Sleep Time: 349, 378, 396

Minutes (left axis): 0, 15, 30, 45, 60, 75, 90, 105, 120

Minutes (right axis): 0, 330, 345, 360, 375, 390, 405, 420, 435

Adapted from: Morin CM, et al. *Am J Psychiatry.* 1994;151:1172-1180.

8

pies in general practice is at least feasible.[13,14] For example, the effectiveness of behavioral strategies in a general practice setting was reported by Espie and associates in a study in which primary care and visiting nurses were trained to administer behavioral interventions, including sleep hygiene education, stimulus control, sleep restriction, relaxation, and CBT, to 139 patients with chronic insomnia during six group meetings at weekly intervals.[14] Clinically meaningful improvements in sleep latency and wake time after sleep onset were noted, with more modest increases in total sleep time. These effects were sustained for 12 months.

However, several approaches to broaden the implementation of general practice–based CBT have been suggested and are being evaluated[15,16]:

- Training of nurse practitioners and physician assistants
- Group therapy formats
- Telephone consultations
- Self-help approaches
- Internet-based treatment.

Nonprescription Agents

■ Antihistamines

Sedating antihistamines (**Table 8.2**) are often used by patients to self-medicate for insomnia because of their wide availability and relatively low cost. According to a National Sleep Foundation survey, 23% of all insomniacs use over-the-counter (OTC) medications for sleep.[17]

The primary active ingredient in OTC sleep aids is a first-generation H_1 antihistamine, whose side effect is sedation. Diphenhydramine, the most commonly used agent, is well absorbed and is widely distributed throughout the body, including the central nervous system (CNS). The peak serum concentration is at about 8 hours and the elimination half-life is about 8

TABLE 8.2 — Selected Nonprescription Agents Commonly Used to Treat Insomnia

Active Agent	Dose (mg)	Onset (min)
Sedating Antihistamines		
Diphenhydramine (Nytol, Sleep-Eze, Sominex)	25-50	60-180
Diphenhydramine [plus Acetaminophen] (Anacin PM, Excedrin PM, Tylenol PM)	25-50 250-650	60-180
Doxylamine (Unisom, others)	25	60-120
Dietary Supplements		
Melatonin (available alone or in combination with various vitamins, minerals, amino acids, and herbs)	1-2	60-120
Valerian (available as a dried root for steeping into tea or as an extract, alone or in combination with various other herbs and vitamins)	300-600	Unknown
Other Agents		
Herbals, alcohol, dietary supplements	—	—

Based on information from: Kupfer DJ, et al. *N Engl J Med.* 1997;336:341-346; Sateia MJ, et al. *Lancet.* 2004;364:1959-1973; Benca RM. In: *Insomnia in Primary Care: A Postgraduate Medicine Special Report.* 2004:23-32; Zhdanova IV. *Sleep Med Rev.* 2005;9:51-65; Brzezinski A, et al. *Sleep Med Rev.* 2005;9:41-50; Hadley S, et al. *Am Fam Physician.* 2003;67:1755-1758.

hours. There is some evidence that this agent can be useful for sleep,[18] yet its effects on sleep have not been well characterized. It may undergo rapid development of tolerance[19] and is associated with daytime sedation. It also has central anticholinergic effects, and its use in vulnerable populations, such as hospital inpatients and the elderly, has also been associated with daytime cognitive impairment, delirium symptoms (eg, inattention, disorganized speech, and altered consciousness), and urinary abnormalities.

Other potential side effects include orthostasis, CNS depression, paradoxic excitement, visual disturbances, tachycardia, dry mouth, urinary retention, and constipation.[20] Therefore, the sedating antihistamines have only a limited role in the management of insomnia.[21]

■ Dietary Supplements and Herbal Agents

Although their use is not regulated by the Food and Drug Administration (FDA), dietary supplements and herbal remedies also enjoy extensive use for sleep disorders owing to a variety of factors, including their widespread availability, lack of prescription requirements, relatively low cost, and the widespread belief that they are safe and have a relatively low abuse risk. These include, among others, melatonin, valerian, kava kava (*Piper methysticum*), chamomille, passiflora, avena sativa, and humulus lupulus.

Melatonin

Melatonin is a neurohormone secreted by the pineal gland (**Figure 8.4**) that plays a major role in regulating circadian rhythm. Its secretion increases at night and is diminished by exposure to light. It is thought to have sleep-wake regulating effects under normal conditions by binding to specific melatonin receptors (MT_1 and MT_2) in the suprachiasmatic nucleus, the brain's "master clock."[22] As melatonin blood levels increase in the evening, there is a gradual decline in alertness and arousal in preparation for sleep. Melatonin receptors are also found throughout the body, but their role, when activated, is currently unclear.

Elevated melatonin levels from either endogenous nocturnal production or exogenous daytime administra-

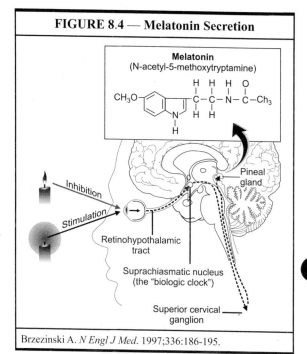

FIGURE 8.4 — Melatonin Secretion

Melatonin
(N-acetyl-5-methoxytryptamine)

Pineal gland

Inhibition

Stimulation

Retinohypothalamic tract

Suprachiasmatic nucleus
(the "biologic clock")

Superior cervical ganglion

Brzezinski A. *N Engl J Med.* 1997;336:186-195.

tion are associated in humans with effects including not only increased sleepiness but also reduced core temperature, increased heat loss, and other generally anabolic physiologic changes.[22] This supports the idea that endogenous melatonin increases nocturnal sleep propensity, either directly or indirectly, via physiologic processes associated with sleep.

Following administration of exogenous melatonin as a dietary supplement, it is rapidly absorbed, with peak levels occurring in 20 to 30 minutes. It has an elimination half-life of 40 to 60 minutes.[23] Sustained-release preparations are also available. Oral doses of 1 to 5 mg result in serum melatonin concentrations that are 10 to 100 times higher than the usual night-time peak within 1 hour after ingestion, followed by a decline to baseline values in 4 to 8 hours.[22]

Behaviorally, the sleep-promoting effects of melatonin are distinctly different from those of common hypnotics and are not associated with alterations in sleep architecture.[24] However, its use in the treatment of insomnia has been limited, perhaps because it appears to have only modest impact primarily in insomnia associated with alterations in sleep phase. One recent meta-analysis of randomized, controlled trials in patients with various types of sleep disorders by Buscemi and colleagues found that compared with placebo, exogenous melatonin decreased sleep onset latency by 11.7 minutes but decreased it by 38.8 minutes in people with delayed sleep-phase syndrome compared with 7.2 minutes in those with primary insomnia.[25]

Another meta-analysis by Brzezinski and coworkers concluded that melatonin treatment significantly reduced sleep-onset latency by 4.0 minutes, increased sleep efficiency by 2.2%, and increased total sleep duration by 12.8 minutes.[26] Since 15 of the 17 studies were performed in healthy subjects or people with no relevant medical condition other than insomnia, the analysis was also done including only those 15 studies. The sleep-onset results were changed to 3.9 minutes, sleep efficiency increased by 3.1%, and sleep duration increased by 13.7 minutes.

On the basis of these analyses, it can be concluded that available evidence suggests that melatonin is not particularly effective in treating most insomnia with short-term use (≤4 weeks); however, some evidence suggests that exogenous melatonin is effective in treating delayed sleep-phase syndrome with short-term use (see Chapter 5, *Common Conditions Associated With Insomnia*).

Melatonin has been shown to have rhythm-altering effects on sleep and wakefulness. Following early evening administration in normal volunteers, it results in a decrease in sleep latency, possibly owing to advance of the sleep-wake rhythm.[27,28] It has also shown benefit in a limited number of studies in various circadian rhythm disorders, such as jet lag,[29] and delayed sleep-phase syndrome.[30] However, melatonin has yielded inconsistent results when used as a hypnotic in other insomnia populations, possibly owing to differences in preparations and dosages utilized, variations in timing of exposure, and other limitations in study methodology. A recent meta-analysis of published melatonin studies concluded that melatonin is not effective in treating most primary or secondary sleep disorders with short-term use.[31,32] Additionally, the report indicated that there is some evidence to suggest that melatonin is effective in treating certain circadian rhythm disorders such as delayed sleep-phase syndrome but no conclusive evidence to indicate that it is effective in alleviating the sleep-disturbance aspect of jet lag and shift-work disorder.

Melatonin's side effects have not been well explored. Although it causes dramatic physiologic effects in species with seasonally regulated physiologies, similar effects have not been described in humans. The risks associated with prolonged use are unknown. Side effects include headache and daytime sedation, and isolated cases of disorientation, seizures, nausea, and dyspnea have been reported, but the frequency of such effects appears to be quite low.[33]

Although melatonin is available without a prescription in various formulations and/or in combination with other dietary supplements, a prescription melatonin receptor agonist, ramelteon, has recently been approved for insomnia by the FDA (see Chapter 9, *Pharmacologic Agents for Insomnia*).

Valerian

Valerian extract, derived from the root of *Valeriana officinalis*, a perennial that grows wildly in temperate areas of the Americas and Europe, has long been advocated and used for promoting sleep but until quite recently, evidence for its efficacy and safety has been solely anecdotal.[34] It contains sesquiterpenes of the volatile oil, including valeric acid, iridoids (valepotriates), alkaloids, furanofuran lignans, and amino acids including GABA, tyrosine, arginine, and glutamine.[21,34-36] Although its soporific mechanism of action is unknown, a recent *in vitro* study showed that valerian and valerenic acid are selective agonists of the dopamine 5-HT$_{5a}$ receptor.[37] However, preparation containing valerian often also contain multiple herbs that are touted to help in sleep. Therefore, interactions between these plant extracts, and/or their synergistic effects, may also play a role.

The typical recommended dose is 400 to 450 mg *V officinalis* root, 30 to 60 minutes before bedtime. It is thought to have anxiolytic, muscle-relaxant, and sleep-promoting properties, yet data regarding efficacy are mixed. For example, Stevinson and Ernst analyzed the results of nine randomized, controlled trials of valerian extract and found the results to be contradictory due to the inconsistency between trials in terms of patients, experimental design and procedures, and methodologic quality.[38]

Nevertheless, one multicenter, randomized, double-blind trial in 202 outpatients with a mean duration of nonorganic insomnia of 3.5 months at baseline found that 600 mg/day of a valerian extract was at least as efficacious as treatment with 10 mg/day oxazepam. Both treatments significantly increased sleep quality compared with baseline ($P < 0.01$).[39]

Although the efficacy of valerian still needs to be determined, its side effects are generally mild. Safety data are scant, yet side effects appear to be rare and mild (gastrointestinal irritation, headache); there are case reports of hepatotoxicity in persons taking herbal products containing valerian. However, its slow onset of effect (2 to 3 weeks) renders it unsuitable for short-term use, although it appears to have beneficial effects on sleep architecture that may make it particularly suitable for long-term use and in the elderly.[40] The treatment duration depends on the specific symptoms of sleep disorder, and herbalists recommend a 2- to 3-week break after a 4- to 6-week period of valerian treatment.

Other Herbs and Supplements

Systematic evidence supporting the use of L-tryptophan, an endogenous amino acid available in a variety of dietary supplements, in the treatment of insomnia is very limited and based on studies in small numbers of patients.[21] Furthermore, there are concerns about its possible toxic effects, specifically eosinophila-myalgia syndrome, particularly when used in combination with certain psychiatric medications.

Kava kava, derived from the root of a plant endogenous to the western Pacific (*P methysticum*), has long been used as a hypnotic and anxiolytic. Although it appears to have a rapid onset of effect and an adequate duration of action, reports of serious hepatotoxicity with this preparation have resulted in its being banned in many countries, and the issuance of a Consumer Advisory from the FDA in 2002.[41]

Summary

In summary, despite their potential advantages, the dietary supplements and herbal remedies suffer from a number of drawbacks, including their lack of strict regulation by the FDA, the paucity of studies of their efficacy and side effects, the lack of definitive data regarding optimal dosages, the unknown potential for interactions with other medications not well investigated, and questions regarding the purity of preparations and the potential for their contamination with other active ingredients.

REFERENCES

1. Kupfer DJ, Reynolds CF 3rd. Management of insomnia. *N Engl J Me*d. 1997;336:341-346.

2. Sateia MJ, Nowell PD. Insomnia. *Lancet*. 2004;364:1959-1973.

3. Benca RM. Behavioral and pharmacologic management options for insomnia. *Postgraduate Medicine Special Report*. Minneapolis, Minn: McGraw-Hill Medical Information Services; December 2004; 23-32.

4. Morin CM, Hauri PJ, Espie CA, Spielman AJ, Buysse DJ, Bootzin RR. Nonpharmacologic treatment of chronic insomnia. An American Academy of Sleep Medicine review. *Sleep*. 1999;22:1134-1156.

5. Morin CM. Psychological and behavioral treatments for primary insomnia. In: Kryger MH, Roth T, Dement WC, eds. *Principles and Practice of Sleep Medicine*. 4th ed. Philadephia, Pa: WB Saunders; 2005:726-737.

6. Morin CM, Culbert JP, Schwartz SM. Nonpharmacological interventions for insomnia: a meta-analysis of treatment efficacy. *Am J Psychiatry*. 1994;151:1172-1180.

7. Murtagh DR, Greenwood KM. Identifying effective psychological treatments for insomnia: a meta-analysis. *J Consult Clin Psychol*. 1995;63:79-89.

8. Chesson AL Jr, Anderson WM, Littner M, et al. Practice parameters for the nonpharmacologic treatment of chronic insomnia. An American Academy of Sleep Medicine report. Standards of Practice Committee of the American Academy of Sleep Medicine. *Sleep*. 1999;22:1128-1133.

9. Perlis ML, Smith MT, Cacialli DO, Nowakowski S, Orff H. On the comparability of pharmacotherapy and behavior therapy for chronic insomnia. Commentary and implications. *J Psychosom Res*. 2003;54:51-59.

10. Jacobs GD, Pace-Schott EF, Stickgold R, et al. Cognitive behavior therapy and pharmacotherapy for insomnia: a randomized controlled trial and direct comparison. *Arch Intern Med*. 2004;164:1888-1896.

11. Morin CM, Colecchi C, Stone C, et al. Behavioral and pharmacologic therapies for late-life insomnia: a randomized controlled trial. *JAMA*. 1999;281:991-999.

12. Vincent N, Lionberg C. Treatment preference and patient satisfaction in chronic insomnia. *Sleep*. 2001;24:411-417.

13. Verbeek I, Schreuder K, Declerck G. Evaluation of short-term nonpharmacological treatment of insomnia in a clinical setting. *J Psychosom Res*. 1999;47:369-383.

14. Espie CA, Inglis SJ, Tessier S, Harvey L. The clinical effectiveness of cognitive behaviour therapy for chronic insomnia: implementation and evaluation of a sleep clinic in general medical practice. *Behav Res Ther*. 2001;39:45-60.

15. Bastien CH, Morin CM, Ouellet MC, et al. Cognitive-behavioral therapy for insomnia: comparison of individual therapy, group therapy, and telephone consultations. *J Consult Clin Psychol*. 2004;72:653-659.

16. Ström L, Pettersson R, Andersson G. Internet-based treatment for insomnia: a controlled evaluation. *J Consult Clin Psychol*. 2004;72:113-120.

17. Ancoli-Israel S, Roth T. Characteristics of insomnia in the United States: results of the 1991 National Sleep Foundation Survey. I. *Sleep*. 1999;22(suppl 2):S347-S353.

18. Rickels K, Morris RJ, Newman H, Rosenfeld H, Schiller H, Weinstock R. Diphenhydramine in insomniac family practice patients: a double-blind study. *J Clin Pharmacol*. 1983;23:234-242.

19. Richardson GS, Roehrs TA, Rosenthal L, Koshorek G, Roth T. Tolerance to daytime sedative effects of H_1 antihistamines. *J Clin Psychopharmacol*. 2002;22:511-515.

20. Agostini JV, Leo-Summers LS, Inouye SK. Cognitive and other adverse effects of diphenhydramine use in hospitalized older patients. *Arch Intern Med*. 2001;161:2091-2097.

21. National Institutes of Health. National Institutes of Health State of the Science Conference Statement on Manifestations and Management of Chronic Insomnia in Adults, June 13-15, 2005. *Sleep*. 2005;28:1049-1057.

8

22. Brzezinski A. Melatonin in humans. *N Engl J Med*. 1997;336: 186-195.

23. DeMuro RL, Nafziger AN, Blask DE, et al. The absolute bioavailability of oral melatonin. *J Clin Pharmacol*. 2000;40:781-784.

24. Zhdanova IV. What Every PCP Should Know: Over-the-Counter Insomnia Treatments. In: *Current Perspectives in Insomnia. Medscape Today*. Available at: http://www.medscape.com/viewarticle/495339. Accessed December 13, 2006.

25. Buscemi N, Vandermeer B, Hooton N, et al. The efficacy and safety of exogenous melatonin for primary sleep disorders. A meta-analysis. *J Gen Intern Med*. 2005;20:1151-1158.

26. Brzezinski A, Vangel MG, Wurtman RJ, et al. Effects of exogenous melatonin on sleep: a meta-analysis. *Sleep Med Rev*. 2005;9:41-50.

27. Cajochen C, Jewett ME, Dijk DJ. Human circadian melatonin rhythm phase delay during a fixed sleep-wake schedule interspersed with nights of sleep deprivation. *J Pineal Res*. 2003;35:149-157.

28. Hughes RJ, Sack RL, Lewy AJ. The role of melatonin and circadian phase in age-related sleep-maintenance insomnia: assessment of a clinical trial of melatonin replacement. *Sleep*. 1998;21:52-68.

29. Petrie K, Dawson AG, Thompson L, Brook R. A double-blind trial of melatonin as a treatment for jet lag in international cabin crew. *Biol Psychiatry*. 1993;33:526-530.

30. Kayumov L, Brown G, Jindal R, Buttoo K, Shapiro CM. A randomized, double-blind, placebo-controlled crossover study of the effect of exogenous melatonin on delayed sleep phase syndrome. *Psychosom Med*. 2001;63:40-48.

31. Buscemi N, Vandermeer B, Hooton N, et al. The efficacy and safety of exogenous melatonin for primary sleep disorders. A meta-analysis. *J Gen Intern Med*. 2005;20:1151-1158.

32. Buscemi N, Vandermeer B, Hooton N, et al. Efficacy and safety of exogenous melatonin for secondary sleep disorders and sleep disorders accompanying sleep restriction: meta-analysis. *BMJ*. 2006;332:385-393.

33. American Family Physician. Available at: http://www.aafp. org/afp/990401ap/1911.html. Accessed December 13, 2006.

34. Hadley S, Petry JJ. Valerian. *Am Fam Physician*. 2003; 67:1755-1758.

35. Wagner J, Wagner ML, Hening, WA. Beyond benzodiazepines: alternative pharmacologic agents for the treatment of insomnia. *Ann Pharmacotherapy*. 1998;32:680-691.

36. O'Hara M, Kiefer D, Farrell K, Kemper K. A review of 12 commonly used medicinal herbs. *Arch Fam Med*. 1998;7:523-536.

37. Dietz BM, Mahady GB, Pauli GF, Farnsworth NR. Valerian extract and valerenic acid are partial agonists of the 5-HT5a receptor in vitro. *Brain Res Mol Brain Res*. 2005;138:191-197.

38. Stevinson C, Ernst E. Valerian for insomnia: a systematic review of randomized clinical trials. *Sleep Med*. 2000;1:91-99.

39. Ziegler G, Ploch M, Miettinen-Baumann A, Collet W. Efficacy and tolerability of valerian extract LI 156 compared with oxazepam in the treatment of non-organic insomnia—a randomized, double-blind, comparative clinical study. *Eur J Med Res*. 2002;7:480-486.

40. Wheatley D. Medicinal plants for insomnia: a review of their pharmacology, efficacy and tolerability. *J Psychopharmacol*. 2005;19:414-421.

41. Kava-containing dietary supplements may be associated with severe liver injury. FDA Consumer Advisory, March 25, 2002. Available at: http://www.cfsan.fda.gov/~dms/addskava.html. Accessed December 13, 2006.

8

9 Pharmacologic Agents for Insomnia

Historical Aspects

Although a variety of substances have been used for the treatment of insomnia since antiquity, bromide, introduced in the mid 1800s, was the first agent specifically used as a sedative hypnotic. Chloral hydrate, paraldehyde, urethan, and sulfonyl soon followed.

Chloral hydrate's chemical structure is distinct from that of the barbiturates and benzodiazepines. Prescribed in doses of 500 to 1000 mg, it has a mean half-life of 4 to 8 hours. It is an effective hypnotic and has a rapid onset of action. Side effects include:

- Gastric irritation
- Unpleasant taste and odor
- Daytime hangover
- Light-headedness
- Malaise
- Ataxia
- Nightmares
- Rarely, paradoxic excitement.

Tolerance develops rapidly, usually within 5 weeks of use. Continued use, especially in large doses, can result in:

- Hypotension
- Arrhythmias
- Myocardial depression
- Physical and psychological dependence
- Hepatic damage.

The lethal to therapeutic ratio is quite narrow, and overdose can result in severe respiratory depression, hepatic damage, hypotension, coma, and death. Rapid discontinuation following chronic use is associated with a withdrawal syndrome characterized by delirium, seizures, and death.[1]

The barbiturates (phenobarbital, secobarbital, butabarbital, amobarbital, and pentobarbital) were introduced in the early 1900s and by the 1960s, accounted for 55% of all hypnotic prescriptions.[2] They produce generalized depression of the central nervous system (CNS), ranging from mild sedation to general anesthesia. Despite their past use as sedative-hypnotic drugs, they have been replaced largely by the much safer benzodiazepine receptor agonists (BzRAs) and melatonin receptor agonists for the treatment of insomnia. Hypnotic doses of barbiturates increase total sleep time, decrease sleep latency, the number of awakenings, and the duration of rapid eye movement (REM) and slow-wave sleep. Tolerance is seen following a few days of administration, and total sleep time may be reduced by as much as 50% after 2 weeks of use. Rapid discontinuation typically leads to rebound effects, including a rebound of REM sleep, associated with increased frequency and intensity of dreaming and nightmares. Barbiturates are associated with residual sedation (hangover) and psychological dependence. Barbiturate overdose, especially when it also involves alcohol, can be fatal.[1]

Categories of prescription medications commonly used for the management of insomnia are listed in **Table 9.1**.

Benzodiazepine Receptor Agonists

Owing to their relatively low risk of fatal CNS depression, the BzRAs have almost completely displaced chloral hydrate and the barbiturates as sedative-hypnotic agents. All agents in this class bind to benzodiazepine recognition site of the γ-aminobutyric

TABLE 9.1 — Pharmacologic Agents Commonly Used for Insomnia

Prescription Agents
- Medications approved for insomnia:
  - Benzodiazepine receptor agonists:
    - Benzodiazepines
    - Nonbenzodiazepines
  - Melatonin receptor agonists
- Medications not approved for insomnia:
  - Sedating antidepressants
  - Anticonvulsants

acid type A (GABA-A) receptor complex and augment the effects of GABA. GABA is the most abundant inhibitory neurotransmitter in the CNS and is thought to mediate a wide variety of clinical effects, including anxiety, cognition, vigilance, memory, and learning, among others.[3] GABA is also the major neurotransmitter of neurons in brain structures thought to be critical for the generation of sleep, such as the ventrolateral preoptic nucleus of the hypothalamus.

GABA-A receptors are widely distributed in the CNS, including in the cortex, basal ganglia, and cerebellum.[4] These receptors contain not only the GABA receptor itself but also a benzodiazepine recognition site and a chloride ion channel. GABA-A receptors are composed of 5 subunits (α, beta, γ, epsilon, and rho, **Figure 9.1**). Most GABA-A receptors are composed of 2 α, 2 beta, and 1 γ subunits. The BzRAs bind to the benzodiazepine recognition site, located at the interface of α and γ subunits.[3] Each of these subunits exists in multiple forms, and different combinations of these forms may yield different pharmacologic properties, although this connection has not been firmly established. Benzodiazepines act with comparable affinity at all GABA-A receptors containing a beta, a gamma-2, and any of 4 α subunits (α 1, α 2, α 3, or α 5). They do not interact with receptor subtypes containing an α 4

171

FIGURE 9.1 — The GABA-A Receptor

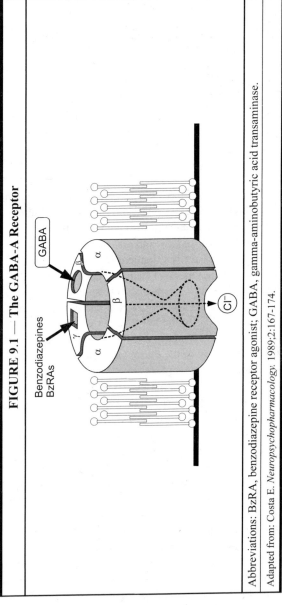

Abbreviations: BzRA, benzodiazepine receptor agonist; GABA, gamma-aminobutyric acid transaminase.

Adapted from: Costa E. *Neuropsychopharmacology.* 1989;2:167-174.

or α 6 subunit. Certain newer hypnotic agents, such as zaleplon and zolpidem, bind more avidly to benzodiazepine receptors containing the α 1 subunit and are, therefore, referred to as selective benzodiazepine receptor agonists (sBzRAs).[5] GABA-A receptors with α1 subunits are thought to mediate the sedative, amnestic, and anticonvulsant effects, whereas those containing α 2 and α 3 subunits are more important for anxiolytic and myorelaxant effects.[6] Nevertheless, the connection between subunit composition and physiologic activity is still under investigation.

The BzRAs that are most commonly used are listed in **Table 9.2** and **Table 9.3**. The first group represents agents that have a benzodiazepine molecular structure. The second group represents agents that are nonbenzodiazepines in structure, and are also sBzRAs.

Various pharmacokinetic properties, including rate of absorption, extent of distribution, and elimination half-life, determine important clinical effects, such as onset and duration of action and the predilection for daytime carryover effects. Some of these clinical effects are summarized in **Figure 9.2**. Sleep latency (SL) is a measure of the time spent falling asleep after going to bed; wake after sleep onset (WASO), the total time spent awake after falling asleep, is a measure of sleep discontinuity during the course of the night; and total sleep time (TST) is a measure of the duration of sleep.

The ideal hypnotic agent would produce benefit in all of these areas without producing daytime residual effects and, in theory, have a pharmacologic profile closely mimicking that seen in **Figure 9.3**. The agent should reach high serum concentrations rapidly so that onset of clinical action can be rapid, a desirable feature for the insomniac whose sleep has a prolonged SL. It should also maintain concentrations above the minimum effective concentration throughout the course of the sleep period in order to maintain sleep throughout the night, a desirable feature for the insomniac with

TABLE 9.2 — BzRAs: Benzodiazepines

Generic (Trade) Name	Dose Range* (mg)	Onset of Action	Half-Life (h)	Active Metabolites
Estazolam (Prosom)	1-2	Rapid	10-24	No
Flurazepam (Dalmane)	15-30	Rapid	47-100	Yes
Quazepam (Doral)	7.5-15	Rapid	27-43	Yes
Temazepam (Restoril)	7.5-30	Slow-intermediate	3.5-18.4	No
Triazolam (Halcion)	0.125-0.25	Rapid	1.5-5.5	No

Abbreviation: BzRA, benzodiazepine receptor agonist.

* Normal adult dose. Dose may require individualization.

Prescribing information: estazolam, flurazepam, quazepam, temazepam, triazolam.

TABLE 9.3 — Selective BzRAs: Nonbenzodiazepines

Generic (Trade) Name	Dose Range* (mg)	Onset of Action	Half-Life (h)	Active Metabolites
Zolpidem (Ambien)	5-10	Rapid	1.5-3.2	No
Zolpidem ER (Ambien CR)	6.25-12.5	Rapid	2.8	No
Zaleplon (Sonata)	5-20	Rapid	1	No
Eszopiclone (Lunesta)	1-3	Rapid	6	No

Abbreviation: BzRA, benzodiazepine receptor agonist.

* Normal adult dose. Dose may require individualization.

Prescribing information: zolpidem, zolpidem ER, zaleplon, eszopiclone.

9

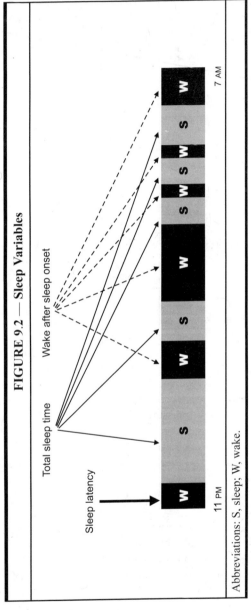

FIGURE 9.2 — Sleep Variables

Abbreviations: S, sleep; W, wake.

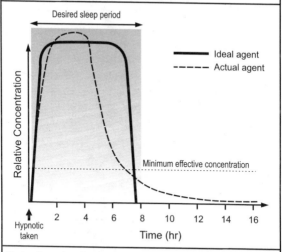

FIGURE 9.3 — Ideal Hypnotic Pharmacokinetic Profile

Desired sleep period

Relative Concentration

—— Ideal agent
- - - - Actual agent

Minimum effective concentration

Hypnotic taken

Time (hr)

Expert Interview. Medscape Psychiatry and Mental Health Web site. Available at: http://www.medscape.com/viewarticle/510414. Accessed October 23, 2006.

sleep discontinuity (repeated nocturnal awakenings resulting in an increase in WASO). Possibly, concentrations of the medication should even increase as the night progresses, in order to compensate for the gradual reduction in the "pressure" to sleep, or the homeostatic factor, as the night progresses. Finally, its concentrations should reach a nadir just prior to the desired awakening time in order to avoid daytime carryover ("hangover") effects, which can cause daytime somnolence, memory impairment, and motor incoordination, among others.

As is evident in **Figure 9.4** and **Figure 9.5**, plasma concentrations of available BzRA hypnotics follow a skewed pattern. In general, their plasma concentrations peak rapidly; therefore, with the possible exception of temazepam,[7] all are effective in reducing SL and

FIGURE 9.4 — Mean Plasma Concentrations of Zaleplon and Zolpidem After Single Doses in 10 Healthy Male Volunteers

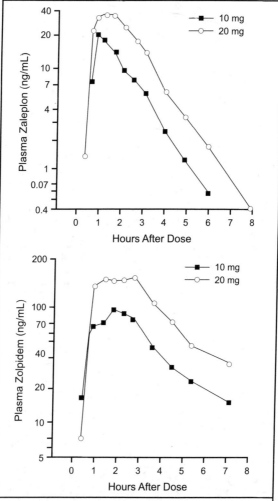

Mean plasma concentrations of zaleplon and zolpidem at corresponding times.

Greenblatt DJ, et al. *Clin Pharmacol Ther*. 1998;64:553-561.

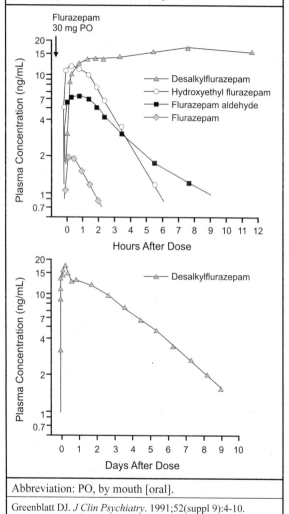

FIGURE 9.5 — Plasma Concentrations of Flurazepam and Metabolites After a Single 30-mg Dose in 18 Healthy Male Volunteers

Abbreviation: PO, by mouth [oral].

Greenblatt DJ. *J Clin Psychiatry*. 1991;52(suppl 9):4-10.

179

are suitable for patients who complain of difficulty in falling asleep upon retiring (**Figure 9.6**).[8] However, plasma concentrations of all hypnotics undergo a gradual reduction over time. As a group, the older BzRAs are effective in increasing TST. They are also effective in maintaining sleep, ie, reducing nocturnal awakenings and increasing TST,[9] although these effects have not been well demonstrated with all of these agents.[10] Therefore, they are also well suited for patients who complain that they awaken repeatedly during the course of the night or who cannot sleep for adequate periods of time. Largely owing to their longer elimination half-life, however (**Figure 9.7**), which results in plasma concentrations that persist for long periods of time, they also have a tendency to produce daytime carryover effects.[8,11-13]

All of the sBzRAs increase TST (**Table 9.4**).[8,14-28] In the case of zaleplon, this feature is limited to the

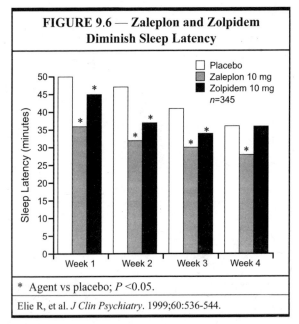

FIGURE 9.6 — Zaleplon and Zolpidem Diminish Sleep Latency

* Agent vs placebo; $P < 0.05$.

Elie R, et al. *J Clin Psychiatry*. 1999;60:536-544.

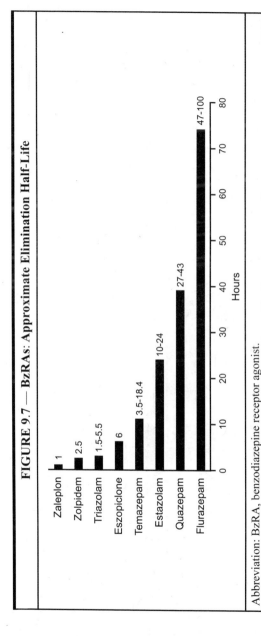

FIGURE 9.7 — BzRAs: Approximate Elimination Half-Life

Drug	Hours
Zaleplon	1
Zolpidem	2.5
Triazolam	1.5-5.5
Eszopiclone	6
Temazepam	3.5-18.4
Estazolam	10-24
Quazepam	27-43
Flurazepam	47-100

Abbreviation: BzRA, benzodiazepine receptor agonist.

Product package inserts (2005). Charney DS, et al. In: *Goodman and Gilman's The Pharmacological Basis of Therapy.* 1996.

9

TABLE 9.4 — Selective BzRAs: Effects on Sleep Variables

Medication	Sleep Latency	Total Sleep Time	WASO
Zaleplon	Yes	Yes*	No
Zolpidem	Yes	Yes	No
Zolpidem ER	Yes	Yes	Yes
Eszopiclone	Yes	Yes	Yes

Abbreviations: BzRA, benzodiazepine receptor agonist; WASO, wake after sleep onset.

* 20-mg dose only.

highest dose of 20 mg.[8,16-28,20] With respect to effects on sleep discontinuity, eszopiclone also diminishes WASO and, therefore, enhances sleep continuity throughout the course of the night.[29] It is the only hypnotic that has been shown to have this effect for as long as 6 months of continuous nightly treatment in a controlled trial (**Figure 9.8**).[20,30] This feature may be due to its relatively long elimination half-life (6 hours) when compared with the other sBzRAs. Zolpidem, on the other hand, which has an elimination half-life of 2.5 hours, has not been shown to enhance sleep continuity.

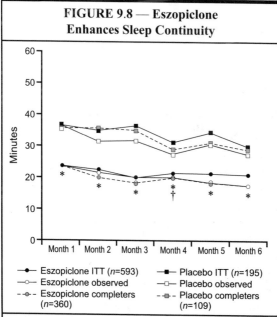

FIGURE 9.8 — Eszopiclone Enhances Sleep Continuity

— ● — Eszopiclone ITT (*n*=593)   — ■ — Placebo ITT (*n*=195)
— ○ — Eszopiclone observed   — □ — Placebo observed
-- ● -- Eszopiclone completers (*n*=360)   -- ■ -- Placebo completers (*n*=109)

Median time wake after sleep onset (WASO) over the treatment period for the intent to treat (ITT) group, observed cases, and completers.

* *P* <0.05 for all comparisons.
† *P* = 0.07 for observed case at month 4.

Krystal AD, et al. *Sleep*. 2003;26:793-799.

183

Zolpidem extended release (ER) was recently introduced. Although the active compound is identical to zolpidem, zolpidem ER consists of a coated two-layer tablet: one layer releases drug content immediately and another allows a slower release of additional drug content, thus providing extended plasma concentrations beyond 3 hours after administration (**Figure 9.9**).[28] This feature imparts zolpidem ER greater efficacy for sleep maintenance than zolpidem following midnocturnal awakenings (**Figure 9.10**)[31]; this was demonstrated in several double-blind crossover studies in younger and elderly patients with chronic insomnia.[14] Zolpidem ER has been shown to diminish sleep discontinuity (decrease WASO) in controlled trials for the first 7 hours during the first two nights and for the first 5 hours after 2 weeks of treatment.[28]

As already mentioned, zaleplon's short half-life of 1 hour makes it suitable for sleep induction, not main-

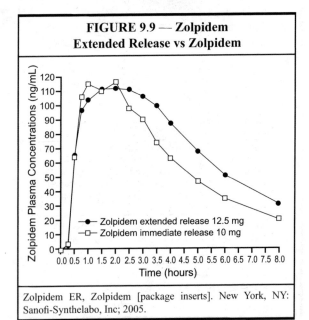

FIGURE 9.9 — Zolpidem Extended Release vs Zolpidem

Zolpidem ER, Zolpidem [package inserts]. New York, NY: Sanofi-Synthelabo, Inc; 2005.

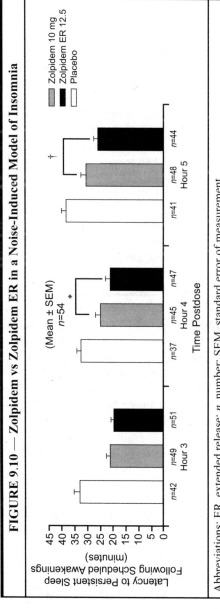

FIGURE 9.10 — Zolpidem vs Zolpidem ER in a Noise-Induced Model of Insomnia

Abbreviations: ER, extended release; *n*, number; SEM, standard error of measurement.

* *P* = 0.0373 vs zolpidem ER.

† *P* = 0.0096 vs zolpidem ER.

Hindmarch I, et al. *Sleep*. 2005;28(abstract suppl):A245-A246. Abstract 0731.

tenance.[19,22] Nevertheless, in the case of discontinuous sleep, it has been shown to be effective in assisting patients in falling back to sleep if administered after awakenings in the middle-of-the-night. If utilized in this fashion, the patient should be advised to remain in bed for a minimum of 4 hours after taking the medication to avoid daytime sedation.[32] Zaleplon's short half-life also increases flexibility regarding the timing of administration for patients who prefer to wait until the last minute, ie, until the need for a hypnotic becomes clearly apparent on any given night. This may make it more conducive for prn use, since patients would take it only if the need for a hypnotic persisted following a period of time in bed.

In the case of the longer half-life medications, prn use is less possible; rather, prophylactic administration in the beginning of the night is necessary to avoid next-day carryover effects. Some have claimed that prn use is ideally suited for the treatment of a disorder such as insomnia that has an episodic longitudinal course, so that the medication can be taken only during an exacerbation of symptoms, thus diminishing the need for hypnotic medications. However, this contention has never been subjected to empiric validation. Since zaleplon produces a short, 4-hour duration of impairment, it is also ideally suited for patients who have reduced sleep times and who have a need to be alert during the day.[33]

As already mentioned, the main adverse effects of the BzRAs are daytime sedation and psychomotor and cognitive impairment. Essentially, these are products of the continuation of the drug's activity during the day. The clinical challenge in using this class of compounds is the identification of a particular medication along the half-life continuum (**Figure 9.7**) at a half-life that will produce maximum efficacy across the night and minimum daytime residual effects. The chronic nature of some patients' insomnia may be necessitate longer

186

treatment. The report of a recent National Institutes of Health (NIH) State of the Science Conference[34] expressed concern regarding the mismatch between the potentially lifelong nature of insomnia and the duration of clinical trials, which, for the most part, has been in the neighborhood of 2 to 5 weeks.

The main concerns in long-term use are tolerance, a decrement in clinical efficacy following repeated use, and rebound insomnia, an escalation of insomnia beyond baseline severity levels following abrupt discontinuation. The latter must be distinguished from a return of symptoms after discontinuation of the medication. Studies of the repeated administration of these agents for 2 to 5 weeks suggest that withdrawal insomnia and rebound phenomena are more pronounced following the administration of higher doses of the benzodiazepine agents that have a short elimination half-life, such as triazolam, than the longer-elimination half-life benzodiazepines and the newer sBzRAs.[35] They are less likely following the administration of long-acting drugs because of the gradual decline in their plasma concentration following discontinuation. Mild and transient withdrawal effects, generally lasting 1 day, have been noted with zolpidem.

More recently, studies of long-term use have been reported. Intermittent treatment over the course of 3 months with zolpidem was conducted, and patients were instructed to take the medication a minimum of 3 and a maximum of 5 pills per week. There was no evidence of tolerance or rebound on nights when the medication was not taken during the entire study (**Figure 9.11**).[36]

Another study utilizing nightly eszopiclone for 6 months in a placebo-controlled design (**Figure 9.8**)[30] revealed no evidence of tolerance during the entire 6-month course or of withdrawal symptoms after rapid discontinuation. In that study, a subset of patients received treatment for an additional 6 months in an

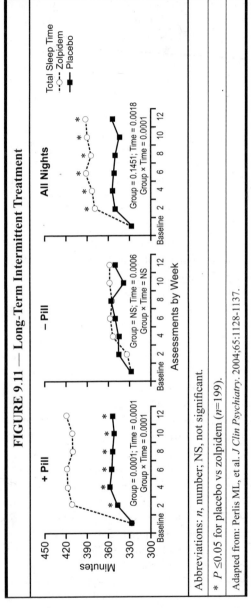

FIGURE 9.11 — Long-Term Intermittent Treatment

Abbreviations: *n*, number; NS, not significant.

* *P* ≤0.05 for placebo *vs* zolpidem (*n*=199).

Adapted from: Perlis ML, et al. *J Clin Psychiatry.* 2004;65:1128-1137.

open-label fashion, and those who had been treated with the medication for 12 months did not exhibit clinically significant withdrawal symptoms after rapid discontinuation of the medication. This study represents the longest controlled use of a hypnotic compound in a clinical trial setting to date. Nevertheless, since withdrawal symptoms can occur in this class of compounds, patients should be carefully monitored following abrupt discontinuation of BzRAs, especially those with shorter half-lives. Even with medications prone to have these effects, the risk of rebound insomnia and withdrawal symptoms can be minimized by utilizing the lowest effective dose and by gradually tapering the dose over the course of a few nights.

Hypnotics should be used with caution in individuals with respiratory depression (eg, chronic obstructive pulmonary disease [COPD] and obstructive sleep apnea syndrome), in the elderly, and in those with hepatic disease, those with multiple medical conditions, and those who are taking other medications that have CNS-sedating properties. They should not be used in pregnant women. Individuals who must awaken during the course of the drug's active period should not take these medications. All are DEA Schedule IV agents and carry a risk of abuse liability (see *Dependence and Abuse* discussion, below). They should, therefore, be used with special caution in individuals with a prior history of alcohol and substance abuse.

Melatonin Receptor Agonists

As noted in Chapter 2, *Normal Sleep*, the sleep-wake cycle represents one of many circadian rhythms that are regulated by an internal biologic clock, which is located in the suprachiasmatic nucleus (SCN) of the anterior hypothalamus. During the course of a typical day, sleep-producing homeostatic factors (sleep debt or sleep pressure) accumulate and intensify in force as the day progresses. In order to maintain the waking state, the SCN produces an opposing wakefulness force, which also intensifies as the day progresses, and which counteracts the homeostatic factor, thus resulting in the maintenance of wakefulness and normal daytime functioning (**Figure 2.9**). Localized to the SCN are melatonin receptors, sites at which endogenous melatonin binds and affects the neuronal output of the SCN. There are two subtypes of such receptors, MT_1 and MT_2, and these are G–protein-coupled receptors.[37] Activation of MT_1 inhibits the neuronal firing rate in the SCN, and MT_2 may play a role in readjustment of circadian rhythm. Throughout the 24-hour cycle, receptor sensitivity fluctuation can be modified by either endogenous melatonin or by heterologous factors

Melatonin receptor agonists act at the MT_1 and MT_2 receptors, and in so doing, are thought to mute the wakefulness force of the SCN, thus allowing the homeostatic factor to dominate, resulting in sleep. Ramelteon is the only melatonin agonist available for clinical use and specifically targets MT_1 and MT_2 receptors with high selectivity.[38] Ramelteon has been shown to reduce sleep latency (**Figure 9.12**).[39] but does not consistently affect TST or WASO.[40] It has also been shown to lack tolerance effects following 5 weeks of continuous administration in controlled trials.[41-43] Additionally, 456 adults and older adults with chronic insomnia did not exhibit rebound insomnia upon discontinuation of ramelteon following 1 year of continuous administration. Three hundred fifty-five patients were adults taking 16 mg of ramelteon, and 101 patients were older adults taking the 8-mg dose.[44]

The most common adverse events that are associated with ramelteon include somnolence, fatigue, and dizziness. It is not recommended for use with fluvoxamine due to a CYP 1A2 interaction. A mild elevation in prolactin levels has been noted in a small number of females and a mild decrease in testosterone values has

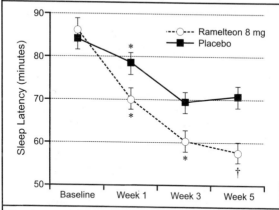

FIGURE 9.12 — Ramelteon Reduced Patient-Reported Time to Fall Asleep in Older Adults With Chronic Insomnia

P values are for comparisons between placebo and ramelteon doses.

* *P* ≤0.01.
† *P* ≤0.001.

Adapted from: Roth T, et al. *Sleep Med*. 2006;7:312-318.

been noted in elderly males, yet the clinical relevance of these changes remains unclear.

Possibly owing to its lack of activity at the GABA receptor, ramelteon does not demonstrate respiratory depression in mild to moderate obstructive sleep apnea syndrome[45] or in mild to moderate COPD.[46] It is DEA nonscheduled and does not carry the risk of abuse liability.

Dependence and Abuse

Hypnotic dependence (addiction) and abuse (an exaggerated desire to obtain the medication in increasing amounts to the exclusion of all other activities)[47] continue to be significant concerns for physicians.

Figure 9.13[48] reviews the relative abuse liability of 19 hypnotic agents. Here, abuse liability is regarded as being a function of both the likelihood that a drug will be abused (used for nonmedical reasons) and the liability of abuse (ie, the untoward or toxic effects of using the drug nonmedically).

The first of these factors, the likelihood of abuse (**Figure 9.13**, white bars), is in turn determined by three factors, namely:

- The degree to which a compound functions as a reinforcer in drug self-administration studies conducted in nonhuman primates
- The extent of drug reinforcement and/or subjective drug liking in humans, as assessed by:
  - Prospective double-blind studies conducted in subjects with histories of drug abuse and assessing drug self-administration, drug choice, or ratings of liking/disliking or positive/negative subjective effects
  - Retrospective questionnaire studies of drug abusers and drug abuse clinicians who rate relative liking or preference for hypnotics based on abusers' histories of exposure to these compounds
- The extent of actual abuse, an estimate of the relative rate of nonmedical use and recreational abuse of the individual hypnotics based on epidemiologic survey data and on case reports of abuse in the medical literature.

The second of these factors, toxicity (**Figure 9.13**, black bars), is determined by:

- The withdrawal severity after termination of chronic supratherapeutic doses of the drug
- The degree of behavioral or cognitive impairment after acute administration of supratherapeutic doses
- The likelihood of death after overdose.

These data suggest that abuse liability of hypnotics is highest for the barbiturate and barbiturate-like medications, intermediate for the BzRAs, low for trazodone, and not present for ramelteon.

Since the risk of abuse or problematic use of hypnotic drugs appears to be more likely in patients with histories of drug or alcohol abuse or dependence, BzRAs should be used in caution or not used at all in patients with such backgrounds.[28] Other groups at risk for the development of problematic hypnotic use include the elderly and patients with chronic pain.[49]

Chronic use of hypnotics has been regarded by many as a measure of abuse. In fact, case reports of physical dependence at appropriate doses of hypnotics following chronic use exist, yet long-term studies examining this question are lacking. Epidemiologic data suggest that the majority of patients use hypnotics for ≤2 weeks[50] and that those who utilize them on a chronic basis do not frequently display dose escalation.[51] Rather, the extent of hypnotic self-administration seems to depend mainly upon the severity of the sleep disturbance on the prior night,[52] indicating a therapeutic pattern of use. Nevertheless, a pattern of long-term use with dose escalation can indicate the potential for hypnotic abuse and such patients should be monitored closely.

Other Prescription Agents

Agents in this class are used as hypnotics but not indicated for this use by the Food and Drug Administration. Nevertheless, they are extensively used for insomnia owing to their low abuse liability, availability of large dose ranges, and low cost. Although these agents may have been studied for their effects on sleep in other conditions complicated by insomnia, only information relative to primary insomnia will be reviewed here.

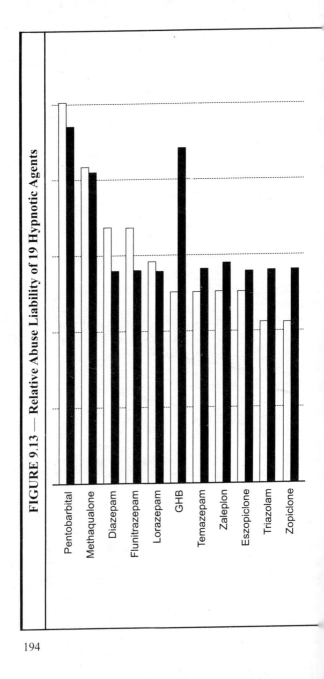

FIGURE 9.13 — Relative Abuse Liability of 19 Hypnotic Agents

Pentobarbital
Methaqualone
Diazepam
Flunitrazepam
Lorazepam
GHB
Temazepam
Zaleplon
Eszopiclone
Triazolam
Zopiclone

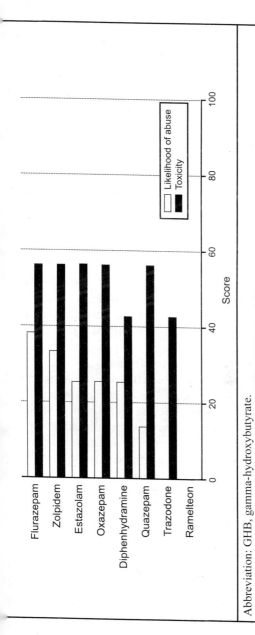

	Likelihood of abuse	
	Toxicity	

Score

Flurazepam
Zolpidem
Estazolam
Oxazepam
Diphenhydramine
Quazepam
Trazodone
Ramelteon

Abbreviation: GHB, gamma-hydroxybutyrate.

Relative abuse liability comprises an assessment of both the likelihood of abuse (white bars) and the toxicity (black bars). Scores show the mean percentage of maximum possible score.

Adapted from: Griffiths RR, et al. *J Clin Psychiatry.* 2005;66(suppl 9):31-41.

9

■ Sedating Antidepressants

These agents are prescribed extensively by physicians[53] despite the fact that there are very limited data on their safety and efficacy in treating insomnia. At appropriate doses, sedating antidepressants have demonstrated efficacy for mood and anxiety disorders. However, in insomnia populations, they are typically utilized at low doses and considered to be subtherapeutic for the treatment of depression or anxiety disorders.

Trazodone is a heterocyclic antidepressant that has an elimination half-life of 5 to 12 hours. It has received little scientific attention as a sleep aid in primary insomnia (reviewed by James and Mendelson in 2004[54]). Walsh and colleagues (1998) reported on a 14-day controlled investigation of trazodone 50 mg, zolpidem 10 mg, and placebo in primary insomniacs.[55] During the first week, both active drugs reduced subjective sleep latency, although trazodone was significantly less effective than zolpidem. By the second week, trazodone's effects were no different from those of placebo.

Doxepin is a tricyclic antidepressant. At doses of 25 mg to 50 mg, it was the subject of a controlled study in 47 subjects with primary insomnia for 4 weeks; it demonstrated an improvement in TST but not in sleep latency.[56] Withdrawal insomnia was evident following abrupt discontinuation. Mirtazapine is a newer antidepressant with an elimination half-life of 20 to 40 hours.[57] It has not been examined in primary insomnia patients.

Therefore, despite their potential advantages, the sedating antidepressants suffer from the major disadvantage of the paucity of available data regarding their effects on sleep and wakefulness in insomnia. Their use is also complicated by daytime sedation and cognitive impairment, anticholinergic effects, weight gain, and drug-drug interactions. The tricyclic antidepressants are also potentially fatal in an overdose.

■ Antiepileptic Drug

The only antiepileptic agent that has been the subject of a formal large-scale investigation for primary insomnia is tiagabine.[58] However, at doses ranging from 2 to 8 mg over the course of 2 nights, it did not have a significant effect on WASO, sleep latency, TST, or the subjective rating of sleep. Its main adverse effects included residual daytime somnolence at the highest dose of 8 mg.

Conclusion

In conclusion, pharmacologic agents play an important role in the management of insomnia. The most salient development over the past few decades has been the development of safer agents. The armamentarium is also beginning to include, for the first time in history, agents with novel mechanisms. The future will likely see a growth in new molecular targets for the treatment of insomnia.

9

REFERENCES

1. Laurence LB, ed. *Goodman & Gilman's The Pharmacological Basis of Therapeutics*. 11th ed. New York, NY: The McGraw-Hill Companies, 2006.

2. Walsh JK, Engelhardt CL. Trends in the pharmacologic treatment of insomnia. *J Clin Psychiatry.* 1992;53(suppl):10-18.

3. Sieghart W, Sperk G. Subunit composition, distribution and function of GABA(A) receptor subtypes. *Curr Top Med Chem.* 2002;2:795-816.

4. Bateson AN. The benzodiazepine site of the GABAA receptor: an old target with new potential? *Sleep Med.* 2004;5(suppl 1): S9-S15.

5. Mendelson WB, Roth T, Cassella J, et al. The treatment of chronic insomnia: drug indications, chronic use and abuse liability. Summary of a 2001 New Clinical Drug Evaluation Unit Meeting Symposium. *Sleep Med Rev.* 2004;8:7-17.

6. Mohler H, Fritschy JM, Rudolph U. A new benzodiazepine pharmacology. *J Pharmacol Exp Ther.* 2002;300:2-8.

7. Heel RC, Brogden RN, Speight TM, Avery GS. Temazepam: a review of its pharmacological properties and therapeutic efficacy as an hypnotic. *Drugs.* 1981;21:321-340.

8. Charney DS, Mihic SJ, Harris RA. Hypnotics and sedatives. In: Hardman JG, Limbird LE, eds. *Goodman and Gilman's The Pharmacological Basis of Therapeutics*. 9th ed. New York, NY: McGraw-Hill; 1996.

9. Greenblatt DJ. Pharmacology of benzodiazepine hypnotics. *J Clin Psychiatry.* 1992;53(suppl):7-13.

10. Rosenberg RP. Sleep maintenance insomnia: strengths and weaknesses of current pharmacologic therapies. *Ann Clin Psychiatry.* 2006;18:49-56.

11. Greenblatt DJ, Divoll M, Harmatz JS, MacLaughlin DS, Shader RI. Kinetics and clinical effects of flurazepam in young and elderly noninsomniacs. *Clin Pharmacol Ther.* 1982;30:475-486.

12. Greenblatt DJ, Harmatz JS, von Moltke LL, et al. Comparative kinetics and dynamics of zaleplon, zolpidem, and placebo. *Clin Pharmacol Ther*. 1998;64:553-561.

13. Roth T, Roehrs TA. A review of the safety profiles of benzodiazepine hypnotics. *J Clin Psychiatry*. 1991;52(suppl):38-41.

14. Moen MD, Plosker GL. Zolpidem extended-release. *CNS Drugs*. 2006;20:419-426.

15. Ambien (zolpidem tartrate) prescribing information. Available at: http://products.sanofi-aventis.us/ambien/ambien.html. Accessed December 13, 2006.

16. Sonata (zaleplon) prescribing information. Available at: http://www.kingpharm.com/uploads/pdf_inserts/Sonata_Web_PI.pdf. Accessed December 13, 2006.

17. Dooley M, Plosker GL. Zaleplon: a review of its use in the treatment of insomnia. *Drugs*. 2000;60:413-445.

18. Hedner J, Yaeche R, Emilien G, Farr I, Salinas E. Zaleplon shortens subjective sleep latency and improves subjective sleep quality in elderly patients with insomnia. The Zaleplon Clinical Investigator Study Group. *Int J Geriatr Psychiatry*. 2000;15:704-712.

19. Fry J, Scharf M, Mangano R, Fujimori M. Zaleplon improves sleep without producing rebound effects in outpatients with insomnia. Zaleplon Clinical Study Group. *Int Clin Psychopharmacol*. 2000;15:141-152.

20. Elie R, Ruther E, Farr I, Emilien G, Salinas E. Sleep latency is shortened during 4 weeks of treatment with zaleplon, a novel nonbenzodiazepine hypnotic. Zaleplon Clinical Study Group. *J Clin Psychiatry*. 1999;60:536-544.

21. Walsh JK, Fry J, Erwin CW, et al. Efficacy and tolerability of 14-day administration of zaleplon 5 mg and 10 mg for the treatment of primary insomnia. *Clin Drug Invest*. 1998;16:347-354.

22. Walsh JK, Vogel GW, Scharf M, et al. A five week, polysomnographic assessment of zaleplon 10 mg for the treatment of primary insomnia. *Sleep Med*. 2000;1:41-49.

9

23. Ancoli-Israel S, Walsh JK, Mangano RM, Fujimori M. Zaleplon, a novel nonbenzodiazepine hypnotic, effectively treats insomnia in elderly patients without causing rebound effects. *Prim Care Companion J Clin Psychiatry*. 1999;1:114-120.

24. Holm KJ, Goa KL. Zolpidem: an update of its pharmacology, therapeutic efficacy and tolerability in the treatment of insomnia. *Drugs*. 2000;59:865-889.

25. Blois R, Gaillard JM, Attali P, Coquelin JP. Effect of zolpidem on sleep in healthy subjects: a placebo-controlled trial with polysomnographic recordings. *Clin Ther*. 1993;15:797-809.

26. Dujardin K, Guieu JD, Leconte-Lambert C, Leconte P, Borderies P, de La Giclais B. Comparison of the effects of zolpidem and flunitrazepam on sleep structure and daytime cognitive functions. A study of untreated insomniacs. *Pharmacopsychiatry*. 1998;31:14-18.

27. Herrmann WM, Kubicki ST, Boden S, Eich FX, Attali P, Coquelin JP. Pilot controlled double-blind study of the hypnotic effects of zolpidem in patients with chronic 'learned' insomnia: psychometric and polysomnographic evaluation. *J Int Med Res*. 1993;21:306-322.

28. Ambien CR [package insert]. New York, NY: Sanofi-Synthelabo, Inc; 2005.

29. Rosenberg R, Caron J, Roth T, Amato D. An assessment of the efficacy and safety of eszopiclone in the treatment of transient insomnia in healthy adults. *Sleep Med*. 2005;6:15-22.

30. Krystal AD, Walsh JK, Laska E, et al. Sustained efficacy of eszopiclone over 6 months of nightly treatment: results of a randomized, double-blind, placebo-controlled study in adults with chronic insomnia. *Sleep*. 2003;26:793-799.

31. Hindmarch I, Stanley N, Legangneux E, Emegbo S. Zolpidem modified-release significantly reduces latency to persistent sleep 4 and 5 hours postdose compared with standard zolpidem in a model assessing the return to sleep following nocturnal awakening. *Sleep*. 2005;28(suppl):A245-A246. Abstract 0731.

32. Corser B, Mayleben D, Doghramji K, et al. No next-day residual sedation four hours after middle-of-the-night treatment with zaleplon. *Sleep*. 2000;23(suppl 2):A309.

33. Doghramji K. The need for flexibility in dosing of hypnotic agents. *Sleep*. 2000;23(suppl 1):S16-S22.

34. National Institute of Mental Health-National Institutes of Health. NIH State of the Science Conference on Manifestations of Management of Chronic Insomnia in Adults. Bethesda, Md; June 13, 2005. *Sleep*. 2005;28:1049-1057.

35. Soldatos CR, Dikeos DG, Whitehead A. Tolerance and rebound insomnia with rapidly eliminated hypnotics: a meta-analysis of sleep laboratory studies. *Int Clin Psychopharmacol*. 1999; 14:287-303.

36. Perlis ML, McCall WV, Krystal AD, Walsh JK. Long-term, non-nightly administration of zolpidem in the treatment of patients with primary insomnia. *J Clin Psychiatry*. 2004;65: 1128-1137.

37. Dubocovich ML, Rivera-Bermudez MA, Gerdin MJ, Masana MI. Molecular pharmacology, regulation and function of mammalian melatonin receptors. *Front Biosci*. 2003;8:1093-1108.

38. Roth T, Stubbs C, Walsh JK. Ramelteon (TAK-375), a selective MT1/MT2-receptor agonist, reduces latency to persistent sleep in a model of transient insomnia related to a novel sleep environment. *Sleep*. 2005;28:303-307.

39. Roth T, Seiden D, Sainati S, Wang-Weigand S, Zhang J, Zee P. Effects of ramelteon on patient-reported sleep latency in older adults with chronic insomnia. *Sleep Med*. 2006;7:312-318.

40. Rozerem (ramelteon). *Physicians' Desk Reference*. Available at: www.pdr.net.

41. Richardson GS, Wang-Weigand S, Zhang J, DeMicco M. Safety assessment of long-term ramelteon in subjects with chronic insomnia. Available at: http://abstractsonline.com/viewer/viewAbstract.asp?CKey={CEF12F4A-46C2-48BF-A85A-AF02429B552C}&MKey={624DA36A-6E6A-40F5-B834-8E6AD1BD1013}&AKey={55ADB755-1C07-404D-8F1E-683043809A66}&SKey={B57FE820-E3B8-474A-B4A4-AFA-BD3E194DA. Accessed December 13, 2006.

42. Roth T, Seiden D, Sainati S, et al. Phase III outpatient trial of ramelteon for the treatment of chronic insomnia in elderly patients. *J Am Geratrics Soc*. 2005;53:S25.

9

43. Erman M, Seiden D, Zammit G, Sainati S, Zhang J. An efficacy, safety, and dose-response study of ramelteon in patients with chronic primary insomnia. *Sleep Med.* 2006;7:17-24.

44. Data on file at Takeda Pharmaceuticals America, Inc; Deerfield, Ill.

45. Sainati S, Tsymbalov S, Demissiel S, Roth T. Double-blind, single-dose, two-way crossover study of ramelteon in subjects with mild to moderate obstructive sleep apnea (poster #480). Presented at: 19th Annual Meeting of the Associated Professional Sleep Societies; June 18-23, 2005; Denver, Colo.

46. Sainati S, Tsymbalov S, Demissiel S, Roth T. Double-blind, single-dose, two-way crossover study of ramelteon in subjects with mild to moderate chronic obstructive pulmonary disease (poster #479). Presented at: Annual Meeting of the Associated Professional Sleep Societies; June 18-23, 2005; Denver, Colo.

47. *Goodman & Gilman's The Pharmacological Basis of Therapeutics.* 11th ed. New York, NY: The McGraw-Hill Companies; 2006.

48. Griffiths RR, Johnson MW. Relative abuse liability of hypnotic drugs: a conceptual framework and algorithm for differentiating among compounds. *J Clin Psychiatry.* 2005;66(suppl 9):31-41.

49. Griffiths RR, Weerts EM. Benzodiazepine self-administration in humans and laboratory animals–implications for problems of long-term use and abuse. *Psychopharmacology (Berl).* 1997;134:1-37.

50. Mellinger GD, Balter MB, Uhlenhuth EH. Insomnia and its treatment. Prevalence and correlates. *Arch Gen Psychiatry.* 1985;42:225-232.

51. Balter MB, Uhlenhuth EH. The beneficial and adverse effects of hypnotics. *J Clin Psychiatry.* 1991;52(suppl):16-23.

52. Roehrs T, Bonahoom A, Pedrosi B, Rosenthal L, Roth T. Disturbed sleep predicts hypnotic self-administration. *Sleep Med.* 2002;3:61-66.

53. Walsh JK. Drugs used to treat insomnia in 2002: regulatory-based rather than evidence-based medicine. *Sleep.* 2004;27:1441-1442.

54. James SP, Mendelson WB. The use of trazodone as a hypnotic: a critical review. *J Clin Psychiatry.* 2004;65:752-755.

55. Walsh JK, Erman M, Erwin CW, et al. Subjective hypnotic efficacyof trazodone and zolpidem in DSM-III-R primary insomnia. *Hum Psychopharmacol.* 1998;13:191-198.

56. Hajak G, Rodenbeck A, Voderholzer U, et al. Doxepin in the treatment of primary insomnia: a placebo-controlled, double-blind, polysomnographic study. *J Clin Psychiatry.* 2001;62:453-463.

57. Timmer CJ, Sitsen JM, Delbressine LP. Clinical pharmacokinetics of mirtazapine. *Clin Pharmacokinet.* 2000;38:461-474.

58. Roth T, Wright KP Jr, Walsh J. Effect of tiagabine on sleep in elderly subjects with primary insomnia: a randomized, double-blind, placebo-controlled study. *Sleep.* 2006;29:335-341.

9

10

Case Studies

Joan T.

This 45-year-old white woman comes to her primary care provider with the chief complaint of feeling tired all the time — for at least the past 6 months, maybe longer. She is asked whether the tiredness is primarily fatigue and a lack of stamina and endurance or whether it is drowsiness and a need to get sleep. She believes it is actually both. She explains that she is easily fatigued as she often has to stop and rest halfway through her household chores, and she had never had to previously. She also states that she has been sleepy during the day; when she sits down to watch television in the afternoon, she becomes drowsy. Taking a nap in the afternoon does not seem to help.

She has been going to bed around 9 PM, "dead tired," which is 2 hours earlier than usual. But oddly enough, even though she is very tired, she has a difficult time falling asleep. When asked what keeps her awake, she does not have an explanation but admits to having some trouble getting settled in bed. She has no worries and says that she has no physical symptoms that keep her awake. Once she gets to sleep, she does sleep through the night but still feels as if she has not gotten a good night's sleep. Her bedroom is otherwise comfortable and quite amenable to sleep. She has never experienced sleep difficulties before, and knows of no one in her family that has. She is asked if her husband has ever remarked about her sleep, specifically whether she snores or has unusual movements in sleep, and she believes that he has noticed nothing of the sort.

- **Medical History**
  - Four pregnancies, three children, one miscarriage; last delivered 6 years ago; husband had vasectomy 5 years previous
  - Seasonal allergies

- **Medications**
  - Over-the-counter (OTC) medication for allergies

- **Medication Allergies**
  - None

- **Social History**
  - Homemaker, part-time work as school aide
  - No alcohol or tobacco use
  - Good diet
  - Until recently, exercised three times per week; now only able to exercise once a week in a limited fashion

- **Family History**
  - Father: age 69; coronary artery disease; hyperlipidemia; hypertension
  - Mother: age 66; obese; total abdominal hysterectomy in late 40s for fibroids
  - Siblings: patient is oldest of three sisters, one younger sister has depression; all else negative

- **Review of Symptoms**
  - Psychiatric inventory normal
  - Heavy menstrual periods for a year, lasting 7 days with first 3 days producing clots
  - Reports heart beating hard when she exerts herself, and momentarily feels light-headed when she gets up too quickly
  - Now admits to and describes weird sensations in her legs when she is watching television at night and has to move them to get comfortable.

She also recalls that their intensity prevents her falling asleep when she is in bed, and she must move her legs in order for the sensations to stop. This gives her temporary relief, but the sensations build up again over the next few minutes so that she has to move again.

■ Physical Examination
- Height, 5' 5"; weight, 133 lb (no recent significant change)
- Blood pressure (BP), 100/70 mm Hg; heart rate (HR), 92; respiration rate (RR), 12; temperature, 97.7°F
- Orthostatic BP, 90/60 mm Hg; HR, 106
- No other remarkable findings

■ Laboratory Tests
- Complete blood count (CBC): hemoglobin (Hb), 11.9, otherwise normal
- Iron (Fe)/total iron-binding capacity (TIBC), transferrin: normal
- Thyroid stimulating hormone (TSH): normal
- Ferritin: 6 (normal: 20-247)

■ Differential Diagnosis
- Iron deficiency
- Anemia, likely secondary to menorrhagia, rule out other causes
- Restless legs syndrome (RLS)
- Other

■ Treatment and Discussion
Given the above information, the patient was advised that the most likely cause of her tiredness was RLS (see also Chapter 5, *Common Conditions Associated With Insomnia*) but probably iron deficiency and mild anemia as well. She was told that her iron stores were low enough to be the cause of the RLS, and

that her iron deficiency and anemia were likely due to menorrhagia. Management included:

- She was advised to take OTC ferrous sulfate 325 mg once a day, increasing eventually to three times daily. She was instructed on precautions and side effects. She was also advised to eat a diet rich in iron. Ferritin levels to be rechecked in 2 months.
- Gynecologic consultation for evaluation and management of menorrhagia
- Specific medication for RLS was left optional, although she was advised to consider temporary use of ropinirole until the condition resolved
- Practice of good sleep hygiene.

In this example, the insomnia was secondary to a treatable condition and addressing the latter was sufficient. It should be noted that iron storage deficiency is sufficient to cause RLS, even in the absence of anemia, microcytosis, and/or deficiency of circulating iron. Levels of ferritin <50 have been shown to be the cause of RLS.[1]

It should also be noted that follow-up is crucial in this patient. Specifically:

- She should be followed via monthly office visits to ensure that her symptoms improve over the ensuing few months. Weekly phone calls should be encouraged since this contact will hopefully increase compliance and favorable results.
- During follow-up, the patient should be given the option of symptomatic treatment of her RLS, and sleep hygiene should be emphasized.
- Her iron studies and hemoglobin should be retested in 2 months to ensure proper rate of rise and return to normal.
- Gynecologic consultation should be followed through to ensure that it is the cause of her iron loss. If this is found not to be the (sole) cause of

her iron deficiency anemia, other causes should be investigated.

- If symptoms do not improve with resolution of her iron deficiency, work-up should continue for her tiredness; during this work-up, she may be considered to have idiopathic RLS and medication to relieve symptoms should be offered.

Marie S.

This 57-year-old African American woman comes to her primary care physician with a chief complaint of headache. Her pain is mostly in the back of her head and neck, and is bilateral. She describes the pain as a tightness and/or pressure. The pain is rarely associated with any other symptoms, except for some nausea when the pain is incapacitating. The headache is constant every day, with varying intensities. She did not note what made the headaches worse (eg, diet, time of day, exercise, weather change). She has been having these headaches for >2 months. OTC analgesics have not provided any relief. On two occasions, the headache evolved into a typical migraine, which she had not experienced for nearly 2 years. These headaches were different: right frontal, throbbing, quite severe (incapacitating), and associated with nausea and light sensitivity. They both occurred upon arising and she had to stay in bed and try to make them go away with OTC agents and sleep. Otherwise, she has not noticed other visual disturbances or neurologic symptoms and denies any recent trauma.

When she was asked about stressors, she began to sob and explained that she was separated from her husband with the intent to divorce. She had become especially upset and despondent over the past few months when she learned that her husband was "getting serious" with another women. Although still able to work as a nurse, she has little energy and motivation to do her job. She stopped taking her daily walks and has lost about 10 pounds due to lack of appetite. In addition, she ceased to participate in some previously enjoyable activities, such as visiting her children and going shopping.

She was asked about her sleep and she reports definite trouble sleeping, which is very bothersome. Although she can fall asleep easily, she awakens after 2 hours, worrying and with her mind racing, then struggles for about an hour to fall back asleep. Furthermore, she awakens at about 4 AM, again unable to fall back to sleep even though she does not need to get up until 6 AM. She has never experienced any problem with sleep, so it is quite upsetting for her. She feels that it adds to her lack of energy and daytime troubled thinking and bad mood. Others noticed that she looks tired. She tried an OTC combination of acetaminophen and diphenhydramine, which helped very little and made her groggy during the day. She has not tried napping as she has no time to do so. No one in her family has any major sleep problems that she knows of, and she has no current bed partner that could also comment on her sleep.

- **Medical History**
  - Never pregnant
  - Obesity
  - Prehypertension
  - Total abdominal hysterectomy with bilateral salpingo-oophorectomy 13 years previous

- **Medications**
  - Currently none; discontinued hormone replacement therapy 3 years previous; OTC vitamin supplements with calcium

- **Social History**
  - Full-time registered nurse at local hospital on permanent day shift
  - Quit smoking 20 years ago; no alcohol; no drugs
  - Caffeine: 2 cups of tea daily, only in the morning; no other sources
  - Recent loss of appetite; discontinued daily walks

- **Family History**
  - Father: deceased at age 78 from stroke
  - Mother: age 79; obese; diabetes mellitus; rheumatoid arthritis; lives in another state with her younger and only sister.

- **Review of Symptoms**
  - Negative other than medical history above

- **Physical Examination**
  - Well-developed, well nourished
  - Tearful, poor eye contact
  - Height, 5' 6"; weight, 188 lb; (body mass index [BMI] = 31.3); lost 10 lb recently
  - BP, 136/88 mm Hg; HR, 84; RR, 14; temperature, 98.0°F
  - All other physical findings within normal limits

- **Mental Status Examination**
  - Sleep disturbance: yes
  - Interest or pleasure: diminished in almost all activities
  - Guilt: some feelings of excessive worthlessness or guilt
  - Energy: fatigue or energy loss nearly every day
  - Concentration: abilities diminished
  - Appetite: weight loss and decreased appetite
  - Psychomotor: some agitation and irritability

- Suicide: no recurrent thoughts of death or suicidal ideation

■ **Differential Diagnosis**
  - Major depressive disorder (MDD)
  - Chronic insomnia comorbid with MDD
  - Headache, most likely tension type, with few migraines
  - Prehypertension

■ **Treatment and Discussion**
The patient is advised that she is suffering from depression with insomnia that goes along with it. She agreed and is ready to do what it takes to get better. She is reassured that with counseling, medication, and a relatively short period of time, her condition should improve and abate. She agrees to see a psychologist but needs to check with her insurance carrier for providers in her area. In addition, she was reassured that her new headaches are most likely of the tension type and she agrees to forego any imaging studies for now.

She adamantly refuses to take any antidepressant because she had heard they can cause weight gain. However, she was receptive to receive treatment for her insomnia.

Sleep hygiene measures are explained and reinforced, and a prescription sleep aid is prescribed.

When choosing a medication for insomnia in patients such as Marie, one can choose from a variety of hypnotic medications (see Chapter 9, *Pharmacologic Agents for Insomnia* for discussion of these agents). Considerations for medication choices should include:

  - *Duration of action of the medication, matching it to the specific characteristics of the patient's insomnia*: For example, agents with the shorter elimination half-life (eg, zaleplon and ramelteon) would be more suitable for patients who primarily have difficulty falling asleep. Agents with a longer elimination half-life (eg, zolpidem ER, eszopiclone) would be more suitable for patients who have difficulty staying asleep during the night.

- *Scheduled nature of the medication*: This is less of a clinical issue, since this patient does not have a history of substance abuse.
- *Long-term usage*: At this point, the patient is not likely to need medication for a long period of time, so this issue is currently moot. The product-insert language regarding long-term use of the most popular sleep medications are less restrictive for zolpidem ER, eszopiclone, and ramelteon.
- *Indication for sleep maintenance*: Of the most popular sleep medications, eszopiclone and zolpidem ER have language that suggests use for sleep maintenance.
- *Prescription coverage*: In this patient's case, she has a copay cost savings for generic medication.
- *Cost*: The patient has a prescription plan.

The better choices for this patient appear to be zolpidem ER and eszopiclone. Based on evidence suggesting benefits of the latter in treating insomnia in patients with MDD, eszopiclone may be an appropriate choice. Marie is prescribed eszopiclone 3 mg taken prior to bedtime and is asked to call in 1 week and return in 2 weeks.

The patient calls back in a week as advised, reporting that she has been following the sleep hygiene measures and taking her medication regularly. As a result, she has been sleeping better with no middle-of-the night awakenings; she has been able to sleep until her alarm goes off at 6 AM. Even though she still feels just as depressed, she is able to function a bit better during the day. She has the side effect of being a bit tired for the first hour that she is up but this is mild. She reports a bit of a metal taste when she first gets up, but it goes away after she brushes her teeth. She reports that she found a psychologist in her insurance network, has seen her once, and seems motivated to continue. She also states that she is now ready to consider taking an antidepressant, as this was also advised by the psychologist. She is given some choices to consider for her office visit in a week.

When seen for her follow-up visit as scheduled, she relays the same information as she did over the phone: still sleeping better but her mood was no better. More information about the selective serotonin reuptake inhibitors (SSRIs) and other antidepressants is provided. She asks for fluoxetine since her copay is the lowest for this. Fluoxetine, initially half of a 20-mg tablet once daily, is prescribed. She is advised to call in 1 week, and return in another 2 weeks. She is also encouraged to continue her psychotherapy sessions.

When she calls 1 week later, she reports still sleeping well and also possibly a little less depressed. During the follow-up visit 1 week later, she appears to be noticeably improved:

- Sleep disturbance: none
- Interest or pleasure: a bit better; restarted walking
- Guilt: less feelings of excessive worthlessness or guilt
- Energy: better
- Concentration: better
- Appetite: improved a bit, weight unchanged
- Psychomotor: less agitation and irritability
- Suicide: no recurrent thoughts of death or suicidal ideation

She is compliant with the medications and reports no new problems. She is asked to continue her current regimen, keep her appointments with her psychologist, and return in 1 month.

When she returns 1 month later as scheduled, she states that she feels close to her old self. Nevertheless, she is advised that optimally, patients with a first episode of MDD should continue the SSRI for 6 months after remission. She also reports that she tried stopping the sleep medication several times but ended up with sleepless nights. She is advised to continue regular use if desired, and when she is ready, she would be instructed on how to wean off of the eszopiclone. She was advised to return in 2 months.

George M.

A 33-year-old white male financial analyst presents to the clinician's office reporting that he has difficulty falling asleep. The difficulty began in his teens, yet was not particularly impactful until he accepted a new position about 6 months ago. This position required him to be to work at 7 AM, making it difficult to sleep later in the morning. He now reports escalating daytime sleepiness with some difficulty concentrating on his work.

The patient states that he intermittently had difficulty falling asleep in college graduate school when he was preparing for exams, but these episodes were self-limited and he did not take any medications to help him sleep. He scheduled his courses such that he would not have to get out of bed earlier than 11 AM. More recently, the patient has had a series of important work-related projects and has kept fairly late hours at the office. He reports coming home by 8:30 PM during the week, eating dinner with his wife, doing some last-minute work on his computer, and getting into bed by 1 AM. Despite feeling tired, the patient reports that he cannot fall asleep until 2 to 3 AM and begins to get frustrated, watching the clock and thinking about his responsibilities of the next day, worrying about the negative impact of his sleeplessness on his daytime performance and health, and feeling tense and upset. Sometimes he begins to watch television or read a magazine in bed if his wife is asleep.

On weekdays, his alarm is set for 5 AM. It is very difficult for him to get out of bed and he feels sleepy all day. On weekends, he is able to sleep in, getting out of bed at 1 PM, and feeling less sleepy during the day. However, he still falls asleep at 2 AM, despite going to bed earlier at times. He denies any daytime nervousness, jitteriness, palpitations, shortness of breath, diaphoresis, or changes in appetite, motivation, or libido; however, he does report considerable daytime irritability. He reports that their relationship with his wife is good but thinks his work schedule might be infringing on his relationship somewhat. His wife denies that the patient snores loudly or demonstrates jerky movements while asleep.

■ **Medical History**
  • Seasonal allergies

■ **Surgical History**
  • Extraction of wisdom teeth 10 years ago

■ **Medication Allergies**
  • Sulfa, which results in rash

■ **Medications**
  • Occasional OTC sinus medication when allergies are bad

■ **Family History**
  • Siblings: one brother, age 28 years, and one sister, age 34 years, both of whom are in good health
  • Father: history of coronary artery disease and coronary artery bypass graft surgery 6 years ago
  • Mother: history of thyroid condition

- ■ **Social History**
  - Lives with his wife of 5 years; no children
  - Does not smoke and drinks occasionally at social events and on weekends
  - Does not use illicit drugs of any kind
  - Drinks 4 to 6 cups of coffee daily, the last one being at 4 PM
  - Works as a financial analyst for a brokerage firm

- ■ **Review of Symptoms**
  - Negative for headache, fever, chills, changes in vision, weight loss or gain, sore throat, heartburn, chest pain, orthopnea, edema, abdominal pain, nausea, vomiting, diarrhea, or constipation

- ■ **Physical Examination**
  - Well-developed, well-nourished man in no acute distress
  - BP, 124/80 mm Hg; pulse, 80; RR, 16; temperature, 97.8°F
  - Head, eyes, ears, nose, and throat: Pupils equally round and reactive to light and accommodation; extraocular muscles are intact. Oropharynx clear without erythema or exudates. Neck: supple with full range of motion. No lymphadenopathy, jugular venous distention or thyromegaly
  - Cardiac: Normal S_1 and S_2; no murmur, rub, or gallop
  - Lungs: Clear to auscultation and percussion
  - Abdomen: Bowel sounds present; soft, non-tender abdomen without mass or hepatosplenomegaly
  - Extremities: No cyanosis, clubbing, or edema; no joint swelling or effusions
  - Skin: Warm and dry; no rash or lesions
  - Neurologic: Mental status—cooperative and oriented ×3 (person, place, and time); intact judgment, above-average insight, functional

10

thinking, and logical speech. Cranial nerves, 2-12 grossly intact. Deep tendon reflexes, + 2/4 at upper and lower extremities bilaterally; negative Babinski's reflexes. Muscle strength, +5/5 in all groups. Sensory, light touch intact. Cerebellar, normal gait; negative Romberg's sign. Psychiatric, normal affect with eye contact

■ **Differential Diagnosis**
  • Hypothyroidism: thyroid function test within normal limits (WNL)
  • Primary ("psychophysiologic") insomnia: tension as bedtime approaches, clock-watching, negative and catastrophic thoughts; all support this diagnosis
  • Major depression: patient does not feel depressed and there is no evidence of anhedonia; Beck depression scale score WNL
  • Obstructive sleep apnea syndrome: no symptoms to support
  • RLS: no symptoms to support
  • Sleep hygiene impairment: caffeine late in the day, excessive caffeine use, delayed bedtimes on weekdays, and delayed awakening times on weekends
  • Delayed sleep-phase syndrome: most consistent with all the facts; lifelong history of delayed bedtime, impairment when the patient is forced to get up early, pattern of delayed bedtime establishes itself when the patient is allowed, such as on weekends

■ **Course of Action**
  • Restrict caffeine to 2 beverages per day and restrict consumption to morning hours
  • Regular bedtime; go to bed at 10 PM on weekdays and weekends, out of bed at 5 AM on weekdays and 6 AM on weekends

- No napping
- Do something relaxing before bedtime
- Come home from work earlier, no working on the computer after 6 PM
- Follow progress with sleep logs

■ Follow-Up Visit in 2 Weeks

- Patient complies with all measures
- Sleep log reveals persistent inability to fall asleep prior to 2 AM, despite keeping of regular morning awakening times
- Sleepiness during day increasing; falling asleep while driving occurs
- Frustration increasing as bedtime approaches; patient has high level of distress

■ Course of Action

- Bright-light therapy in the morning; ask patient to either go outdoors at 5 AM for 1 hour, or recommend exposure to bright artificial light, full spectrum no UV, 10,000 lux, for 1 hour in the morning on weekends and weekdays
- Begin cognitive behavioral therapy; weekly sessions with behavioral nurse specialist, who addresses thoughts of catastrophic things and misperceptions in 30-minute sessions
- Follow progress with sleep logs

■ Follow-Up Visit in Another 2 Weeks

- Log shows earlier falling-asleep times of midnight to 1 AM
- Continued adherence to regular awakening times
- Bright-light exposure daily in the morning
- Daytime sleepiness decreasing; improved ability to focus on work duties
- Outlook improving, less distressed
- Wife reports less moody at home

■ Long-Term Recommendations

- Maintain morning regular awakening times of 5 to 6 AM on all days, regardless of social activities
- Ongoing exposure to bright light as much as possible
- Avoid work after 6 PM; adhere to sleep hygiene measures
- Call physician if sleep times become delayed

Mark K.

This 20-year-old college sophomore comes to see his primary care physician concerning his trouble concentrating. He had shared this concern with a fellow student who then told him that he had the same problem and was diagnosed with attention-deficit/hyperactivity-disorder (ADHD). Therefore, the patient is concerned about whether he has ADHD. He also reports problems with sleep. He notes that he studies until midnight and then goes to bed. However, he will toss and turn, unable to get to sleep until 1 or 2 AM. This has been going on for months, ever since his returning from winter break.

As a result, he feels tired during the day. He bought an OTC aid (containing a sedating antihistamine) and it provided little help. Moreover, it made him feel groggy in the morning and he had more trouble functioning in class. Despite trying to catch up on weekends by sleeping until 11 AM, this did not help relieve his tiredness. He reports never having trouble sleeping in the past. His mother experiences insomnia, and he recalls her taking a sleep medication every night. Addressing his chief complaint, he admits to a history of inattention and disruptive behavior throughout his previous schooling. With the patient's permission, a phone call to his parents confirms this. They add that he has always had problems with organization and they have been frustrated by his lack of responsibility with household chores. They do not recall many problems in school until he reached the 9th grade when his grades started to dip. They add that he never studied, and believe he would have done better if he was not so lazy and would have applied himself.

- **Medical History**
  - Unremarkable other than above
  - No adverse reactions to medications

- **Social History**
  - Nonsmoker; denied drug and alcohol use
  - Caffeine; a few colas a day, none after dinner

- **Family History**
  - Parents and two younger brothers are in good health, except middle sibling recently started to experience similar attention and distractibility problems in the 11th grade.
  - The patient mentioned that his mother has always been a "poor sleeper"

- **Review of Symptoms**
  - Brief psychiatric inventory unremarkable
  - Patient has 7 out of 9 positive answers for inattention, 6 out of 9 for hyperactivity/impulsivity

- **Physical Examination**
  - Well-developed, typically dressed, pleasant and cooperative
  - No remarkable findings
  - Persistent rapid bouncing of one foot on the floor

- **Differential Diagnosis**
  - ADHD
  - Chronic insomnia, likely comorbid with ADHD
  - Delayed sleep-phase syndrome (DSPS)

- Chronic insomnia, possibly comorbid with an as yet undiagnosed psychiatric problem

■ Treatment and Discussion

The patient meets all of the DSM-IV-TR criteria for ADHD. He is given information on this and information on medications currently indicated for it. This is also relayed to the parents. He is advised that his sleep problem could be due to several possibilities, and that it could be related to the ADHD. Due to time constraints, the patient is asked to return after a few days and to keep a sleep log.

When the patient returns a few days later, he and his parents have agreed that long-acting methylphenidate is best for him. They have read all of the material on it, and are aware of its pros and cons, as well as the necessary precautions. He is advised to take the medication every morning at the same time. He is now also instructed in sleep hygiene measures, namely:

- Try to go to bed when drowsy, eg, 1 AM, and to get up at the same time every day, eg, 8 AM, even on weekends.
- Try to keep the room dim and quiet during bedtime, asking his roommate to cooperate.
- Read something pleasant and noneducational for 15 to 20 minutes before trying to go to sleep.
- Move the clock out of view.
- Try to take a half-hour to 1-hour nap in the afternoon; he felt that the dorm was quiet enough for this to be possible.

The patient returns 1 week later reporting some improvement in his ability to concentrate, but he feels it could be better. He is given explicit instructions on titrating the medication upward. He also notes improvement in daytime sluggishness. He attributes the latter to regular afternoon napping. However, he is still struggling with falling asleep despite trying to

222

follow the advice previously given. At this point, there are several possible courses of action:

- Further reinforcement of sleep hygiene measures
- Referral to the school psychologist for cognitive behavioral therapy for his insomnia (see Chapter 8, *Behavioral Strategies and Nonprescription Agents*)
- Prescribing a sleep medication.

In this case, all three are employed. Considerations for medication choice involve:

- Patient only has sleep-initiation insomnia and does not need help with sleep maintenance
- Patient is a college student, where misuse and abuse of scheduled substances is more of a concern
- Difficulty initiating sleep, which may be appropriately addressed with a short half-life hypnotic agent
- Possible need for long-term use
- Cost and insurance constraints.

He is prescribed the melatonin receptor agonist, ramelteon 8 mg, to be taken one-half hour before going to bed.

The patient returns 1 week later as advised, reporting continued use of methylphenidate as directed, which is "working perfectly." He is following the sleep hygiene instructions more often than not. He has also met once with the school psychologist and continues to do so weekly. He is particularly happy that he is now able to fall asleep at a reasonable hour, getting into bed at 1 AM and falling asleep in about half an hour. He also notes his daytime functioning to be good. He is advised to continue taking the sleep medication for a full month and to return after that time. He is to return in 2 weeks for refilling his ADHD medication and follow-up. The patient returns a few days past 2 weeks, stating that he had run out of the sleep medication a few days prior and is still sleeping fine. He is taking the methylphenidate as directed. This is renewed, and the sleep medication is not. He is advised to return in another month but to call sooner if the insomnia recurs.

Charles D.

This 52-year-old man comes in for a comprehensive medical evaluation (complete physical). He has no specific complaints.

■ **Medical History**
  - Status, postappendectomy
  - Medications: none

■ **Social History**
  - Lifelong nonsmoker, rare, modest alcohol use
  - No exercise
  - Accountant, lives with wife; their two children moved away

■ **Family History**
  - Father: died at age 65 from myocardial infarction; may have had hypertension
  - Mother: age 79, alive and well
  - Siblings: patient has one older brother, health unknown

■ **Review of Symptoms**
  - All essentially negative except for sleep. He states that "I've had trouble sleeping all my life." He also relates that ever since he was a teenager, he has struggled to fall asleep, taking an hour or so. This worsens when life stresses increase and at times even causes him to awake

in the middle of the night or wake up too early. He normally goes to bed at 11 PM, falls asleep sometime after midnight, and wakes up at 5 AM without an alarm, even though he does not have to leave for work until 7:30 AM. He considers himself to be a light sleeper, since any minor thing will wake him up. He never feels totally refreshed during the day but never feels drowsy and cannot take naps. He has never mentioned his sleep problems to any medical provider since none asked, and he did not think it was important enough to bring up. He has tried a few OTC sleep aids in the distant past but only rarely since he does not believe in taking drugs in order to sleep. His mother told him that he mirrored his father's personality of being "hyper" and sleeping poorly.

- Psychiatric inventory normal

■ Physical Examination

- Height, 5' 8", weight, 152 lb (no recent significant change)
- BP, 140/90 mm Hg; HR, 88; RR, 12; temperature, 98.2°F
- General appearance: healthy-looking, well-dressed, somewhat jittery
- No other remarkable findings.

■ Laboratory Tests (obtained prior to visit)

- Chemistry profile, CBC, TSH, prostate-specific antigen (PSA), urinalysis, all normal
- Lipid panel:
  - Triglycerides: 224 mg/dL
  - Total cholesterol: 194 mg/dL
  - Low-density lipoprotein (LDL): 118 mg/dL
  - High-density lipoprotein (HDL): 28 mg/dL

■ Differential Diagnosis
- Primary insomnia
- Hyperlipidemia, mixed type
- Hypertension suspected

■ Treatment and Discussion

Given the preceding information, the patient is advised that he most likely has primary insomnia, a chronic condition for which some people are more vulnerable than others. He is told that his insomnia could be affecting his daily functioning, and he agrees that he should be feeling better during the day and would invite suggestions at improving his sleep to improve his waking periods.

Alternatives, including cognitive behavioral therapy, OTC herbal aids, and prescription medications, are discussed. He is not interested in the former two but is willing to consider a prescription medication since he has seen ads on television that described their benefits, but most importantly because his mother is doing so well on zolpidem. He is advised that eszopiclone and zolpidem ER would be equally good choices, but he chooses zolpidem.

Considerations for medication choices include:
- Patient has sleep-initiation insomnia and impairment in the duration of sleep
- Patient is motivated to take zolpidem, and this is an appropriate medication for him
- Cost and insurance.

Zolpidem 10 mg is prescribed. He is advised to take the medication every night at 11 PM and to make sure he has a good 6 hours in bed. He restates that he never uses alcohol and has no intention of using it now, with or without the sleep medication. He is instructed to call if any problems occur.

The patient returns in 2 weeks as advised. He remarks eagerly that he has never slept as well as he has in the past 2 weeks. He falls asleep well before midnight (he believes it is around 11:30 PM) and sleeps soundly, deeply, and continuously. He did not realize how poorly he had been functioning during the day until the past 2 weeks demonstrated how well he felt. He is getting at least 6 hours of sleep and reports no side effects. He asks for a 90-day prescription since his pharmacy plan allows him to use a mail-away pharmacy for maintenance medications. However, he is told this not preferred as yet; he is given a prescription for a 30-day supply and asked to return in another month.

The patient returns in a month as planned. He states that he is still sleeping well, although at times he finds himself waking up early again. He is given the option of switching to the long-acting version of zolpidem, and he agrees. His prescription is changed to zolpidem ER 12.5 mg. He is advised to phone in 1 week with a report. The patient does so and reports better sleep, waking up now at 6 AM, which suits him just fine. He once again asks for a 90-day prescription and is advised that this would be considered at his next appointment in 2 months.

The patient returns in 2 months and continues to express his elation at how well he is sleeping and how well he continues to feel during the day. He is still going to bed at 11 PM and waking up at 6 AM. He is adhering with all of the instructions and precautions. A 90-day prescription with no refills is given, and he is advised that he should return every 3 months for follow-up.

REFERENCE

1. Silber MH, Richardson JW. Multiple blood donations associated with iron deficiency in patients with restless legs syndrome. *Mayo Clin Proc.* 2003;78:52-54.

INDEX

Note: Page numbers in *italics* indicate figures;
page numbers followed by t refer to tables.

11

11

11

11

11

242

11

11

11

Rozerem (ramelteon). See *Ramelteon*.

11

11

11